Essential Oil Recipes:

ONE DROP AT A TIME

Revised Edition

Like us on Facebook for contests and updates
www.facebook.com/EverydayOilSolutionsInc

Buy our books on Amazon or our Etsy Shop
www.etsy.com/shop/EverydayOilSolutions

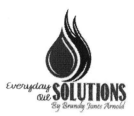

Compilation by Brandy Jones Arnold
Cover Design by Brandy Garison

Table of Contents

Abbreviation Guide

- EO   Essential Oil
- CO   Carrier Oil
- RB   10 ml Roller Bottle
- LB   Pound
- t   Teaspoon
- T   Tablespoon
- C   Cup
- Oz   Ounce

Frequently Asked Questions

Are all essential oils created equally?

There are vast differences in the quality of essential oils available on the market. We are selective when it comes to what we bring into our homes, what we put on our children's plates, and what products we use to care for our families. These same research-driven principles should also apply to how we select a brand of essential oil. Not all essential oils are created equally. Purity and quality matter, as do the service and reputation of the company you choose to buy from. Your goal when deciding which brand(s) to use should be to find unadulterated, quality essential oils and to purchase them from a company you trust.

Why does the purity of essential oils matter?

You will be breathing your essential oils, in some cases ingesting them, and most of the time applying them topically. Skin is the body's largest organ, accounting for more than 10% of body mass. Essential oils easily absorb through the skin, as do chemicals and toxins. Most of us are aware that common household chemicals found in cleaners, beauty products and plastics have been known to be responsible for various illnesses, including but not limited to cancer, developmental defects in children and attention deficit hyperactivity disorder.

Essential oils are a means to a healthier, chemical-free lifestyle. When you make this transition, be sure that you are using pure and unadulterated essential oils that offer you therapeutic benefits and improve your health and well-being. Inferior quality, adulterated oils are not likely to produce therapeutic results and can in fact be dangerous to users in terms of toxicity and allergic reactions as well.

What should I look at when selecting an essential oil company?

Ideally you want a company that has been in the Aromatherapy field for an established number of years and carries a strong ethical reputation, that is owned by an essential oil specialist, and will provide batch specific MS/GC spec reports and MSDS sheets. You want the company to oversee the day to day processes and operations closely to monitor cultivation, harvesting and distillation and verify purity at every critical junction, as well as a company that can attest to the fact that they use sustainable farming practices, non-GMO seeds, and essential oils as pesticides, versus chemicals. When you are making the decision on which essential oil brand to choose, you need to be able to call the company and ask about these issues, and receive reasonable answers. In addition, you need to know:

- Do they provide complete distill or first distill?
- Do they distill and bottle their own oils or outsource?
- Do they test each batch for purity? If so, is the testing done in-house or by third party?
- Do they own their own farms? If so, are they open to the public to tour?
- Do they recommend that you not ingest their oils?

How exactly are essential oils used?

EO's are used in 3 simple ways:

- Aromatically – Therapeutic benefits of essential oils are gained by inhalation. This includes inhalation from the bottle, via a diffuser or aromatic jewelry piece, or even simply from a drop placed on the hands cupped around your nose and mouth. This is one of the most powerful and effective ways to use essential oils.
- Topical Application – This involves putting essential oils on the skin, your largest organ, either neat (direct application with no carrier oil) or with a CO (carrier oil). This is an excellent way to get powerful oils into the blood stream quickly. They enter our circulatory system within approximately 20 seconds, and penetrate every cell in our bodies within 20 minutes. Oils can be diluted and applied to a specific area of the body including the temples, spine, jawline, wrists, feet, reflex points and chakras.
- Ingestion – Many users of quality, unadulterated essential oils choose to ingest oils for greater absorption and overall wellness support. Some oils, labeled as dietary supplements, are ingestible. However, proper brand selection is a MUST, as ingesting low quality or adulterated essential oils can be toxic. Most essential oils found at health food stores and discount chains say, "Not for internal use." Even if a bottle says, "100% Pure Essential Oil," it could still be cut with chemical fillers. Individual essential oil research is imperative also, as every oil is unique, thus usage guidelines will vary greatly amongst oils. Certain oils such as Wintergreen, Rue, and Mugwort should never be ingested. Peppermint should not be used on children under 30 months, and Cassia is a dermal sensitizer and could irritate nasal membranes if inhaled directly from the bottle.

What is a carrier oil (CO)?

A carrier oil is a vegetable oil such as coconut oil or sweet almond oil that can be used to dilute essential oils, and in effect act as a vehicle to "carry" the essential oil into your body in an efficient and comfortable manner. This does not reduce the impact of the essential oil and prevents waste. Common carrier oils include coconut, grapeseed, jojoba, sweet almond and castor oil. Refer to individual essential oil bottle labels for dilution recommendations for each oil. Some oils can be applied neat, or without dilution. Please exercise caution when choosing a CO if you have any type of nut allergy.

What should I look for when choosing a carrier oil?

Much of this is personal preference, and you want the most nourishing, freshest carrier oils possible. Many factors play a role in determining which oil you choose, including processing method, shelf life, and intended location and purpose of application. According to the National Association for Holistic Aromatherapy, some carrier oils are better suited for certain purposes than others. For example, sweet almond oil can help relieve itchiness and dry skin. Avocado oil is excellent for regenerative skin care and mature skin. Calendula aids in soothing insect bites and is anti-inflammatory, while tamanu can help promote healthy scar formation (www.naha.org). Kim Harris Mullins does an excellent write up on the subject titled "Carried Away: A Guide to Carrier Oils for Essential Oils." It can be found on her blog at https://oilsandspoils.blog/

Are certain carrier oils more likely to clog pores than others?

Yes. You will find a Comedogenic (pore-clogging) chart for various carrier oils located on page 90.

What should I do before using an essential oil?

A patch test! To perform a patch test, apply 1-2 drops of essential oil to a patch of skin, preferably to the bottom of the feet. Watch that area over the course of 1-2 hours for any reaction, but most, if any, reactions will occur within 5-10 minutes.

Where should I use my essential oils?

Essential oils can be used in a variety of locations, including the temples, wrists, neck, spine, bottom of feet, stomach, muscles, jawline, chakras, etc. Essential oils are also highly effective when applied to the many reflex or vita flex points located throughout the body, primarily on the hands, feet and spine. NEVER use essential oils directly in your eyes OR inside of your ears. Concerning sensitive skin, such as mucous membranes and genitalia, usage is not recommended.

Are essential oils safe to ingest?

This is a very controversial topic, and knowledge of the fact that the market is flooded with fragrance oils, synthetics and adulterated oils diluted with toxins explains why. Dr. Kurt Schnaubelt comments on the controversy surrounding the topic and states, "those engaged in the manufacture and distribution of adulterated oils, knowing about the added or synthetic chemicals, will warn against ingesting oils," *(Schnaubelt, Kurt, Ph.D. The Healing Intelligence of Essential Oils. The Science of Advanced Aromatherapy. Rochester, VT: Healing Arts Press, 2011, p 132.)* Dr. Schnaubelt continues to say, "Ingested essential oils…reach the liver very quickly where they are metabolized and eliminated. It is advantageous to ingest an essential oil only if the metabolic intermediates produced during elimination create a desired therapeutic effect and safety parameters are favorable."

It is an individual decision to which there is no clear-cut answer. To decide if ingesting an oil is right for you, let common sense prevail. What is your research, knowledge and personal experience with the oil at hand? Do you trust that your oils are unadulterated? The FDA has approved some essential oils for internal use and given them the designation GRAS (Generally Regarded as Safe for internal consumption); is the oil regarded as GRAS? Would potential benefit from ingesting this oil outweigh any potential risk associated with this oil?

Cautionary note: If you decide to ingest an oil, it is necessary that you read labels and look for the wording "fit for consumption" or "for dietary usage." Ensure you trust the brand of essential oils you choose are pure, unadulterated, and fit for ingesting. If you have any doubt about the quality and origin of your essential oils, DO NOT INGEST THEM. Before ingesting any Generally Regarded as Safe (GRAS) essential oils, ensure that you first test for reactions by diluting 1 drop of essential oil in 1 tablespoon of coconut oil or other carrier oil; closely monitor for adverse reactions.)

How often can essential oils be applied?

Proper usage should be indicated on each essential oil label. Always follow label instructions. Essential oils are very potent – always start low and go slow, and adhere to the mantra "more is sometimes less." According to the *Essential Oil Desk Reference*, when applying oils for the first time, do not apply more than two single oils or blends at once. In most cases 1-2 drops are sufficient – but depending on the essential oil, you can gradually build up to 3-4 uses per day *(Essential Oils Desk Reference, Sixth Edition. Lehi, UT: Life Science Publishing, 2015, p 34.)*

What if I experience skin discomfort or irritation while applying the oil?

If a reaction occurs, stop using the essential oil and apply a carrier oil to the affected area. Never use water to attempt to flush the oil off the skin, as the water won't adhere to the oil and remove it. Only another oil will "grab" the essential oil and remove it, ensuring relief as quickly as possible. Before attempting to use the essential oil again, be sure to perform a patch test and dilute with carrier oil.

If a rash should result, it is possibly a sign of detoxification. While using essential oils, it is imperative to drink plenty of water to encourage the release and removal of toxins. Toxins present in petrochemical based soaps, skin care products, detergents, deodorants and perfumes may trigger detox reactions. These chemicals are present in many forms in our homes. Personally, I have embarked on a mission to eradicate as MANY chemicals in my household as I can by replacing store bought products with chemical-free alternatives I can easily make with recipes found in this book.

What is a "hot oil"?

Hot oils, when applied to the skin, can cause a hot or burning sensation. Always use CO with hot oils. If a reaction DOES occur, stop using the essential oil and apply a carrier oil to the affected area. Common hot oils include:

- Basil
- Cassia
- Cinnamon Bark
- Clove
- Cumin
- Eucalyptus
- Lemon Myrtle
- Lemongrass
- Mountain Savory
- Orange
- Oregano
- Peppermint
- Thyme
- Wintergreen

Are certain essential oils photosensitive?

Some EOs, especially citrus oils, contain natural molecules that can react with sunlight and cause a reaction, including but not limited to rash, burn, blistering and dark pigmentation. It is best that these oils are worn under the clothing, out of the path of direct sunlight. Again, please read all labeling before usage. Oils known to cause photosensitivity include Angelica, Bergamot, Bitter Orange, Cumin, Grapefruit, Lemon, Lemon Verbena, Lime, Mandarin, Orange, Tangerine and Tagetes.

What supplies will I commonly use with my essential oils?

Common containers to have on hand include 2, 4, 8 and 16 oz glass spray bottles, 5 and 10 ml glass dropper bottles, 10 ml roller bottles (preferably with stainless steel roller balls), size '00' empty vegetable capsules, and miscellaneous glass jars that range in size.

Carrier oils good to have on hand include coconut oil, fractionated coconut oil, sweet almond oil, grapeseed oil, vitamin e oil, argan oil and jojoba. Other ingredients you will frequently need include shea butter, cocoa butter, vegetable glycerin, distilled water, Epsom salt, sea salt, baking soda, witch hazel, white vinegar, honey and vanilla extract.

A few of our favorite places to shop for supplies:

- ✓ www.bulkapothecary.com
- ✓ www.abundanthealth4u.com
- ✓ www.gotoilsupplies.com
- ✓ www.etsy.com/shop/ChemistryCo
- ✓ www.amazon.com

Are essential oils safe for use on children?

Concerning the decision to use essential oils on yourself or your child, always perform due diligence, do your research, ask advice, but foremost, consult your Physician. Many essential oils are appropriate for use on children. The safest place to apply essential oils to children is the bottom of their feet, due to thicker skin. The feet also correlate to the vita flex points mentioned previously.

Due to the sensitive nature of a child's skin, dilution is always necessary. Carefully follow dilution instructions found on essential oil bottles. When in doubt, dilute 1:30. Keep oils out of the reach of children, as you would for any product intended for therapeutic use. D. Gary Young, ND, in his book entitled *Essential Oils Integrative Medical Guide,* recommends that essential oils should not be given as dietary supplements to children under 6 years of age. Young further states "essential oils rich in Menthol (such as Peppermint) should not be used on the throat or neck area of children under 30 months of age." (*Young, D. Gary. Essential Oils Integrative Medical Guide. Building Immunity, Increasing Longevity, and Enhancing Mental Performance with Therapeutic-Grade Essential Oils. Lehi, UT: Life Science Publishing, 2013, p 37.*)

The following Dilution Chart is recommended for Children:

6 months – 2 Years = Dilute 4x the label recommendation

2 Years – 5 Years = Dilute 3x the label recommendation

5 Years – 10 Years = Dilute 2x the label recommendation

Debra Raybern is the author of *Gentle Babies,* "which combines two decades of professional knowledge with tried-and-true techniques and first-hand testimonials." (*Reybern, Debra. Gentle Babies, Essential Oils and Natural Remedies for Pregnancy, Childbirth, Infants and Young Children. Revised Fifth Edition. Bartlesville, OK: Growing Healthy Homes, LLC, 2014, p 15.*) It is an easy to follow guide for expecting and new mothers. She states that for babies under age 2, oils to "be cautious of or avoid altogether...include Eucalyptus, Basil, Juniper, Peppermint, Hyssop and Wintergreen."

Raybern continues the opinion concerning oils safe to use on children include, but are not limited to:

- Bergamot
- Cedarwood
- Cypress
- Frankincense
- Geranium
- Ginger
- Lavender
- Lemon
- Marjoram
- Melaleuca Alternifolia (Tea Tree)
- Orange
- Roman Chamomile
- Rose Otto
- Rosemary
- Rosewood
- Sandalwood
- Thyme
- Ylang Ylang

Are essential oils safe to use during pregnancy?

As with any medical condition, prior to use of essential oils, seek the advice and guidance of a competent, trained health care advisor. Debra Raybern is again my source for this question in her well-respected book *Gentle Babies*. Her research indicates that "often the following are mentioned in aromatherapy guides as oils to avoid during pregnancy: Basil, Birch, Calamus, Cassia, Cinnamon Bark, Hyssop, Idaho Tansy, Lavandin, Rosemary, Sage, Tarragon, and Wintergreen" as well as the blends that contain these oils *(p 14.)*

The *Quick Reference Guide for Using Essential Oils* by Connie and Alan Higley indicates that Angelica, Carrot Seed, Cedarwood, Chamomile, Cistus, Citronella, Clary Sage, Clove Bud, Cumin (Black), Cypress, Davana, Fennel, Laurel, Marjoram, Mountain Savory, Myrrh, Nutmeg, Peppermint, Rose, Rosemary, Spearmint, Tarragon, Vetiver and Yarrow should be used with caution during pregnancy. Again, always do your research, and exercise due diligence *(Higley, Connie & Alan. Quick Reference Guide for Using Essential Oils. Spanish Fork, UT: Abundant Health, 2014, p 278.)*

How can I use essential oils to enhance my spiritual life?

We love to hear this question! This book focuses on recipes that address your physical, stress and emotional responses. For information on essential oils in your spiritual life, we recommend the work of Rev. Dr. Katy E. Valentine at Agápe Spiritual Care. With her Ph.D. in Biblical Studies, Rev. Dr. Valentine has a solid background in spiritual care and diverse areas of interest that intertwine her background with her passion for oils. Areas of expertise include clearing chakras, anointing oils and oils of the Bible, and oils used in meditation. You can connect with her at www.agapespiritualcare.com or her Etsy shop www.etsy.com/shop/agapespiritualcare, where she has chakra blends available made from unadulterated essential oils, as well as a Meditation CD I highly recommend.

How do I use this book?

This recipe book was created as a general guideline to give you safe direction, incentive and courage to make your own creations and have some fun along the way! Everyone is unique. Due to that fact, essential oils and these recipes will have individual results. With certain issues, you might need to tweak and modify, possibly removing one oil, or adding a few more drops of another. "Higher dosages of essential oils should only be utilized after you have gradually built the necessary experience with such doses, enabling you to know which essential oils you can tolerate in this fashion," *(Schnaubelt, Kurt, Ph.D. The Healing Intelligence of Essential Oils. The Science of Advanced Aromatherapy. Rochester, VT: Healing Arts Press, 2011, p 129.)*

The best advice I can give you is to make notes, either in the margins of the pages or in the Notes Section found at the back of the book. Jot down your findings and what works best for you! Don't let lack of an essential oil deter you from trying a recipe. Many essential oils have similar key constituents and can be substituted with other oils to obtain results. When in doubt, the *Essential Oil Pocket Reference* by Life Science Publishing is an excellent resource for finding information on essential oils, history, usage information, and medical properties.

Don't be afraid of trial and error, don't hesitate to do your own research, and don't give up on a recipe too soon. Sometimes results take a bit of time. But after a few weeks, if you have not seen significant results, don't be afraid to try something new!

Ailments: Respiratory

Cold and Flu User Guide

A BLEND OF CLOVE, LEMON, CINNAMON BARK, EUCALYPTUS RADIATA AND ROSEMARY is your first line of offense and defense concerning your wellness. According to legend, this blend dates back centuries and is popular today because of its effectiveness at boosting the immune system and is anti-bacterial, anti-infectious, anti-septic and anti-viral. Most essential oil companies include a similar blend in their starter kits. If you already own this blend, substitute it throughout the book when "Antibacterial Blend" is called for. If you do not, here is a simple recipe to create a blend very similar on your own:

Antibacterial Blend – Dropper Bottle

40 drops Clove

35 drops Lemon

20 drops Cinnamon Bark

15 drops Eucalyptus Radiata

10 drops Rosemary

In a 5 ml dropper bottle, combine all ingredients. Do not apply this recipe neat, it must be diluted prior to using.

Offensively: Dilute this recipe 1:8 (1 drop Blend and 4 drops CO) and put on the bottom of your feet daily to boost immunity.

Defensively: If you are feeling under the weather

- Dilute this recipe 1:4 and apply on the bottom of your feet every few hours
- Diffuse 6-8 drops three times a day
- Adults can put 1 drop inside cheek and under tongue every few hours
- Dilute 1:4 and rub on the outside of the neck for a sore throat
- Put 2 drops in a tablespoon of honey and swallow

LAVENDER is great for congestion and stuffy noses. Apply it neat (undiluted) on the bridge of your nose and the bottom of your feet. For a runny nose, rub under nostrils.

MELALEUCA ALTERNIFOLIA (Tea Tree) can be diluted 1:1 and applied on the outside of the throat when sore. To help with earaches, dilute 1:1 and circle around the outside of the ears. Put 1 drop on a cotton ball, and place lightly in the outer ear, being careful not to get essential oils inside the ear canal. Melaleuca Alternifolia should not be used in children under 6 years of age.

PEPPERMINT is great for congestion and fever. For congestion, dilute 1:8 drops and rub over sinuses and chest. For fever, dilute 1:8 and apply to back of neck, down spine, under armpits, behind knees, around navel, and on bottom of feet. Continue to repeat every 15 to 30 minutes or until fever breaks.

MYRTLE, FIR OR GOLDENROD can be rubbed diluted on the chest or diffused to help with a hacking cough or respiratory congestion.

LEMON can be diffused to help a cough. Put a drop or two in water and drink several times a day to help cleanse your system and stimulate the immune system. To help with drainage, Lemon can be diluted 1:8 and applied behind ears and down the jawline to lymph nodes.

Fever – Single Application

1 drop Peppermint
8 drops CO
Mix ingredients in hand and apply under armpits, down spine and on bottom of feet. Wait 10 minutes and reapply if needed. May also dilute and use Lemon as a substitute.

Cold and Flu Fighter – Capsule

2 drops Antibacterial Blend [Recipe on page 19]
2 drops Lemon
1 drop Oregano
1 drop Frankincense
Add essential oils to a size '00' empty vegetable capsule, top with CO and take orally.

Flu Buster – RB

8 drops Antibacterial Blend [Recipe on page 19]
6 drops Oregano
6 drops Melaleuca Alternifolia
Top with CO. At the first sign of flu, or exposure to flu, apply to bottom of feet every two hours.

Immunity Support for Cold and Flu Season – Diffuser

2 drops Peppermint
5 drops Antibacterial Blend [Recipe on page 19]

Sore Throat Version #1 – Single Application

1 drop Antibacterial Blend [Recipe on page 19]
1 drop Lemon
1 drop Peppermint
Combine all in 1 teaspoon of Honey or a shot glass of water. Gargle and swallow. Repeat every 3-4 hours. Roll Daily Immunity Booster [Recipe on page 33] on bottom of feet every 2 hours as needed, or daily as a preventative measure.

Sore Throat Version #2 – Single Application

2 drops Lemon
1 drop Oregano
Combine all in 1 teaspoon of honey or a shot glass of water. Gargle & swallow. Repeat every 3-4 hours. Roll Daily Immunity Booster [Recipe on page 33] on bottom of feet every 2 hours as needed, or daily as a preventative measure.

Antibacterial Throat - Spray

10 drops Antibacterial Blend [Recipe on page 19]
5 drops Lemon
5 drops Frankincense
3 T Distilled Water

2 t local Honey

1 t Vodka

Add all to 2 oz glass spray bottle. Spray two squirts into back of throat as needed for relief.

Cough Version #1: Dry Cough – Diffuser and Single Application

2 drops Eucalyptus Globulus

2 drops Thyme

2 drops Lavender

Diffuse these oils, and/or dilute with 12 drops CO and apply to chest. Afterwards, cup hands, place over nose and mouth, and breathe deeply.

Cough Version #2: Cough with Mucus – Diffuser and Single Application

2 drops Eucalyptus Globulus

2 drops Thyme

2 drops Melaleuca Alternifolia

Diffuse these oils, and/or dilute with 12 drops CO and apply to chest. Afterwards, cup hands, place over nose and mouth, and breathe deeply.

Cough Syrup – Jar

5 drops Lemon

5 drops Peppermint

5 drops Lavender

5 drops Frankincense

½ C local Honey

Add honey to a 4 oz glass jar. Add essential oils and thoroughly combine. You can take a tablespoon of this every 2-3 hours.

Cough Drops with Honey and Lemon

10 drops Lemon

1 C Honey

1 T Apple Cider Vinegar

Optional: Lollipop Sticks and Candy Mold

Pour honey and apple cider vinegar into a saucepan. Bring mixture to a boil and allow it to reach 300°F, stirring constantly so it doesn't stick. Once it reaches 300°F, remove from heat. After about a minute, add Lemon and stir well. Have a greased cookie sheet or candy molds ready. Allow the mixture to cool just a bit until the honey is slightly less runny. Using a big spoon, drop small amounts into the cookie sheet or into the candy molds, inserting lollipop sticks if you would like. Allow to cool at room temperature until hard, then wrap individually in wax paper or store in an airtight container.

Chest Rub Version #1: Expectorant – Jar

5 drops Ravintsara

5 drops Eucalyptus Globulus

5 drops Wintergreen

5 drops Peppermint
5 drops Tangerine
1 C Coconut Oil
Heat coconut oil in a double boiler over low-medium heat until melted. Remove from heat, cool slightly, and add essential oils, stirring well. Pour into an 8 oz jar and let stand until firm. Rub on chest and throat as needed, breathing deeply while doing so.

Chest Rub Version #2: Decongestant – Jar

10 drops Lemon
8 drops Eucalyptus Globulus
6 drops Cypress
6 drops Peppermint
4 drops Melaleuca Alternifolia
1 C Coconut Oil
Heat coconut oil in a double boiler over low-medium heat until melted. Remove from heat, cool slightly, and add essential oils, stirring well. Pour into an 8 oz jar and let stand until firm. Rub on chest and throat as needed, breathing deeply while doing so.

DisInfect Me! Tea Version #1 – Single Application

1 drop Lemon
1 drop Antibacterial Blend [Recipe on Page 19]
1 drop Frankincense
1 drop Peppermint
Add all essential oils to a mug of hot water or your favorite organic herbal hot tea. Use local honey and sweeten to taste. Drink as often as needed, breathing deeply from the mug as you do so.

DisInfect Me! Tea Version #2 – Single Application

2 drops Lemon
2 drops Antibacterial Blend [Recipe on Page 19]
Add all essential oils to a mug of steaming hot water or your favorite organic herbal hot tea.
Use local honey and sweeten to taste. Drink as often as needed, breathing deeply from the mug as you do so.

Sniffles – Diffuser

5 drops Antibacterial Blend [Recipe on page 19]
1 drop Lemongrass

Sinus Cleaning Trio – Diffuser

3 drops Lemon
3 drops Peppermint
3 drops Eucalyptus Globulus

Sinus Infection – Vapor

2 drops Oregano
2 drops Peppermint
1 drop Melaleuca Alternifolia
1 drop Lemon
1 C Water

In a ceramic mug, add water and heat in the microwave to a boil. Carefully remove the mug from the microwave, let it cool slightly, add essential oils, and stir well. Drape a towel over your head while leaning over the mug and inhale vapors. Repeat several times per day or as often as needed.

Respiratory Support for Spring and Summer Version #1 – Diffuser

3 drops Lavender
3 drops Lemon
3 drops Peppermint

Respiratory Support for Spring and Summer Version #2 – Diffuser

4 drops Eucalyptus Radiata or Globulus
3 drops Melaleuca Alternifolia
1 drop Lemon

Allergy Trio – RB

3 drops Lemon
3 drops Lavender
3 drops Peppermint

Add all to an empty RB and top with CO. For seasonal respiratory relief, apply daily along back of neck, throat, and bottom of feet plus inhale directly for added relief.

Allergy Trio – Capsules

5 drops Lemon
5 drops Lavender
5 drops Peppermint

Add essential oils to a size '00' empty vegetable capsule, top with CO and take orally.

Pollen Be Gone – RB

5 drops Roman Chamomile
5 drops Cypress
5 drops Peppermint
5 drops Lavender

Add all to an empty RB and top with CO. For seasonal respiratory relief, apply daily along back of neck, throat, and bottom of feet plus inhale directly for added relief.

Bath Salts for Nasal Congestion and Sinus Infection – Jar

2 drops Eucalyptus Radiata

3 drops Rosemary
2 C Epsom Salt
1 C Baking Soda
In a large bowl, thoroughly combine Epsom salt and baking soda. Add essential oils and stir well. Pour in a 24 oz glass jar. Add 1 cup to running bath water using the hottest tolerable water temperature. Soak 20-30 minutes. Makes enough for 3 baths.

Shower Vapor Cups – Jar

4 drops Peppermint
4 drops Eucalyptus Globulus or Radiata
3 C Baking Soda
Muffin Tin
Muffin Paper Liners
Line the muffin tin with your muffin papers. In a medium bowl, mix baking soda with enough water to make a paste. Spoon baking soda mixture into muffin papers and let them dry in a cold oven for 12-18 hours. Once hardened they are ready to use. Store the discs in an airtight container. When ready to use, remove one from the container and add 4 drops of Peppermint and 4 drops of Eucalyptus on top of the disc and place in your shower for vapors.

Ailments, Digestive

Stomach Bug Regimen

Rub 2 drops each Peppermint, Ginger and Juniper diluted in a teaspoon of CO clockwise on stomach to relieve nausea and help cleanse your body of the bug. Wipe excess on bottom of feet. You can also add 2 drops of Peppermint and Ginger to a size '00' empty vegetable capsule, top with CO and take orally.
Diffuse Antibacterial Blend [Recipe on page 19]
Use Antibacterial Blend, diluted 1:4 and apply on the spine and bottom of feet.
Dehydration is usually a result of the stomach bug. Drink water as often as you can, and add 1-2 drops of Lemon to your water to help detox your body daily.

Bellyache Buster/Hiccups – RB

8 drops Peppermint
8 drops Tarragon
4 drops Cypress
Top with CO. Apply clockwise over the stomach and on chest and throat if there are esophageal issues.

Motion Sickness and Nausea – RB

10 drops Peppermint
8 drops Ginger
2 drops Lemon

Top with CO. Apply to wrists, temples, behind the neck and bottom of feet. (Helpful hint: If traveling by sea, bring Peppermint on the boat and inhale from the bottle if feeling nauseous at any point.)

Cramps – Capsule

3 drops Basil
1 drop Peppermint
1 drop Ginger
Add essential oils to a size '00' empty vegetable capsule, top with CO and take orally.

Too Much Fun the Night Before! Bath Salts – Jar

10 drops Eucalyptus Globulus
5 drops Juniper
2 C Epsom Salt
¼ C Baking Soda
¼ C Kosher Salt
In a large bowl, thoroughly combine Epsom salt, baking soda and kosher salt. Add essential oils and stir well. Pour into a 24 oz glass jar. Add 1 cup to running bath water using the hottest tolerable water temperature. Soak 20-30 minutes. Makes enough for 3 baths.

Ailments, Pain

Headaches – RB

20 drops Peppermint
Top with CO. Rub on temples, top of forehead, brain stem and back of neck. (Helpful hint: You can also layer a few drops of Copaiba for more severe headaches.)

Headache Buster for Sinus Headaches – RB

drops Peppermint
drops Wintergreen
drops Idaho Balsam Fir
drops Lavender
drops Frankincense
Top with CO. Rub on temples, top of forehead, brain stem and back of neck. (Helpful hint: You can also layer a few drops of Copaiba for more severe headaches.)

Migraine Tamer – RB

drops Peppermint
drops Basil
drops Marjoram
drops Frankincense
drops Lavender

Top with CO. Rub on temples, top of forehead, brain stem and back of neck. (Helpful hint: You can also layer a few drops of Copaiba for more severe headaches.)

Migraine Tamer – Diffuser

3 drops Frankincense
2 drops Peppermint
1 drop Lavender
1 drop Marjoram

M Bomb for Pain – Capsule

3 drops Frankincense
3 drops Copaiba
3 drops Idaho Balsam Fir
Add essential oils to a size '00' empty vegetable capsule, top with CO and take orally.

M Bomb Cream for Feet – Jar

12 drops Frankincense
12 drops Copaiba
12 drops Idaho Balsam Fir
½ C Coconut Oil
½ C Shea Butter
Optional: 10 drops Plai and 6 drops Peppermint
Heat shea butter and coconut oil on double boiler until melted. Let cool in fridge approximately 30-60 minutes until barely firm. Whip with electric mixer until light and airy for approximately 10 minutes, then add essential oils. Combine thoroughly. Store in 8 oz glass jars, makes approximately 16 oz.

Muscle Pain or Headache – RB

5 drops Idaho Balsam Fir
4 drops Copaiba
4 drops Peppermint
4 drops Wintergreen
2 drops Helichrysum
1 drop Clove
Top with CO. Roll onto areas of discomfort as needed.

Body Ache and Relaxation Bath Salts – Jar

15 drops Lavender
2 C Epsom Salt
1 C Baking Soda
In a large bowl, thoroughly combine Epsom salt and baking soda. Add essential oils and stir well. Pour into a 24 oz glass jar. Add 1 cup to running bath water using the hottest tolerable water temperature. Soak 20-30 minutes. Makes enough for 3 baths.

Back Pain Bath Salts – Jar

6 drops Peppermint
4 drops Eucalyptus Globulus or Radiata
4 drops Rosemary
3 drops Lavender
1 C Epsom Salt
1 C Dead Sea Salt (can use additional Epsom Salt if you do not have Dead Sea Salt)
1 C Baking Soda
In a large bowl, thoroughly combine Epsom salt and baking soda. Add essential oils and stir well. Pour into a 24 oz jar. Add 1 cup to running bath water using the hottest tolerable water temperature. Soak 20-30 minutes. Makes enough for 3 baths.

Pain Cream – Jar

8 drops Peppermint
7 drops Eucalyptus Globulus
7 drops Wintergreen
7 drops Black Spruce
5 drops Rosemary
1 C Coconut Oil
Optional: Add 10 drops Lemongrass, Copaiba or Idaho Balsam Fir if needed for more effectiveness. Add coconut oil to mixer and blend until light and airy. Add in essential oils and mix well. Store in an 8 oz glass jar. (Helpful hint: This may melt when room temperature is above 76°F, but will firm up again once cool. For faster firming if melted, place jar in the refrigerator.)

Pain Version #1 – RB

5 drops Lemongrass
5 drops Peppermint
5 drops Wintergreen
3 drops Copaiba
Top with CO. Roll onto areas of pain and tension.

Pain Version #2 – RB

3 drops Plai
4 drops Copaiba
4 drops Lemongrass
2 drops Peppermint
Top with CO. Roll onto areas of pain and tension.

Pain and Regenerative Blend – RB

drops Marjoram
drops Lemongrass
drops Wintergreen
drops Palo Santo

2 drops Lavender
Top with CO. Good for injuries and tendon/ligament or cartilage regeneration.

Massage Therapist Muscle Pain – RB

6 drops Palo Santo
4 drops Peppermint
4 drops Lemongrass
2 drops Wintergreen
2 drops Basil
2 drops Marjoram
Top with CO. Use liberally over sore muscles and joints.

Inflammation, Strong Blend – RB

6 drops Cistus
5 drops Lemongrass
4 drops Copaiba
3 drops Helichrysum
3 drops Oregano
3 drops Thyme
2 drops Myrrh
Optional: 4 drops Ravintsara (for inflammation due to infection)
Optional: 4 drops Vetiver (for a relaxant)
Optional: 4 drops Palo Santo (for regeneration)
Top with CO and apply several times daily as needed.

Fibro Pain Cream – Jar

10 drops Peppermint
10 drops Plai
8 drops Copaiba
8 drops Lemongrass
5 drops Wintergreen
5 drops Marjoram
1 C Coconut Oil
Mix well in an 8 oz glass jar and apply as needed to area of discomfort.

Sciatic Pain – RB

6 drops Idaho Blue Spruce
5 drops Idaho Balsam Fir
3 drops Copaiba
3 drops Clove
3 drops Rosemary
Top with CO. Roll onto areas of pain and tension. This is a great muscle, joint and tendon/ligament soother.

Arthritis Pain – Jar

12 drops Dorado Azul
10 drops Frankincense
8 drops German Chamomile
8 drops Wintergreen
8 drops Idaho Balsam Fir
½ C Shea Butter
½ C Coconut Oil
Heat shea butter and coconut oil on double boiler until melted. Let cool in fridge approximately 30-60 minutes until barely firm. Whip with electric mixer until light and airy for approximately 10 minutes, then add essential oils. Combine thoroughly. Store in 8 oz glass jars, makes approximately 16 oz.

Bursitis Technique – Single Application

5 drops Marjoram
3 drops Wintergreen
3 drops Cypress
Apply Marjoram (relieves joint pain/soothes nerves) with equal amount of CO to affected area. Wait 5 minutes, then apply Wintergreen (anti-inflammatory/analgesic) with equal amount of CO. Wait 6 minutes, then apply Cypress (improves circulation/reduces swelling) with equal amount of CO. Optional: Can layer Copaiba afterwards for added relief.

Bursitis Blend – RB

5 drops Dorado Azul
5 drops Marjoram
5 drops Wintergreen
4 drops Cypress
Top with CO. Roll onto areas of pain and tension.

Ailments, Skin

Burns – Single Application

Apply Lavender neat (no dilution) to area of discomfort.

Nosebleeds – Single Application

drops Cypress
Put Cypress on the inside of each forearm. There are two big veins there, and that is one of the fastest ways to get oils into the bloodstream. Will possibly take two applications, but should stop the nosebleed quickly.

First Aid – Spray

10 Melaleuca Alternifolia
10 Eucalyptus Radiata

10 Lemon
½ t Sea Salt
8 T Witch Hazel

Mix the essential oils and sea salt in a 4 oz glass spray bottle, swirling to combine. Top with witch hazel. Shake well before use. Clean all cuts and abrasions thoroughly, then spray the area with First Aid Spray. Afterwards, you may want to cover the area with sterile gauze to which you have applied 3 drops of Lavender. Repeat 2-3 times daily.

Ouch! Oil – RB

8 drops Melaleuca Alternifolia
6 drops Lavender
6 drops Frankincense

Top with CO. Relief for cuts, bumps, bruises, burns and skin issues. If skin is open or bleeding, do not apply RB directly to wound as it may contaminate your RB. For small children see Dilution Chart. Can be used for:

Skin issues Apply directly to affected skin.
Pinkeye Apply around eye socket and down bridge of nose being careful NOT to get in eyes.
Ear infections Apply all around ear. Do not drop oil directly in the ear. May put a drop on a cotton ball, fold over and place gently in outer ear.

Ouch! Oil for Itchy Skin, Rashes, Eczema – RB

5 drops Lavender
5 drops Roman Chamomile
4 drops Melaleuca Alternifolia
3 drops Frankincense
3 drops Rosemary

Top with CO. Apply as needed to areas of discomfort.

Itch Be Gone – Spray

10 drops Lavender
10 drops Frankincense
10 drops Melaleuca Alternifolia
6 T Witch Hazel
2 T Aloe Vera Gel

Combine witch hazel, aloe vera gel and essential oils in a 4 oz glass spray bottle. Mix well. Spritz on skin as needed for soothing the skin due to itching, bug bites, etc.

Minty Cool Sunburn – Spray

32 drops Lavender
24 drops Peppermint
1 C Witch Hazel
½ C Aloe Vera Gel
¼ C Fractionated Coconut Oil

¼ C Distilled Water

1 t Vitamin E Oil

Combine all ingredients in a 16 oz glass spray bottle. Shake well before use. Spray liberally on skin as needed when you have experienced too much sun exposure. (Helpful hint: Storing this mixture in the refrigerator or ice chest until ready to use provides an extra chill to help cool you down on a hot day!)

Lavender Aloe Sunburn – Spray

30 drops Lavender

10 drops Peppermint

10 drops Melaleuca Alternifolia

1 C Aloe Vera Gel

½ C Fractionated Coconut Oil

½ C Witch Hazel

1 t Vitamin E Oil

Combine all ingredients in a 16 oz glass spray bottle. Shake well before use. Spray liberally on skin as needed when you have experienced too much sun exposure.

Eczema Lotion – Jar

12 drops Lavender

12 drops Palmarosa

drops Melaleuca Alternifolia

¼ C Sweet Almond Oil

½ C Shea Butter

½ C Coconut Oil

Heat shea butter, coconut and sweet almond oil in a double boiler until melted. Remove from heat and add essential oils, stirring well. Pour into a 10 oz glass jar and let stand until firm.

Whipped Eczema Cream – Jar

drops Lavender

drops Geranium

drops German Chamomile

¼ C Shea Butter

¼ C Coconut Oil

Heat shea butter and coconut oil in a double boiler until melted. Remove from heat, cool slightly and add essential oils, mixing well. Place bowl in the refrigerator and let cool for approximately 30-60 minutes, until firm but not hardened. Once firm, you can use the eczema cream, but if you whip with an electric mixer for approximately 5-10 minutes, it yields a creamier consistency. Whipping the mixture yields approximately 8 oz.

Rosacea Be Gone – Dropper Bottle

drops Lavender

drops Melaleuca Alternifolia

drops German Chamomile

3 drops Geranium
Fractionated Coconut Oil
Top essential oils with coconut oil in a 10 ml dropper bottle. Apply twice daily to affected area thoroughly after washing your skin.

Psoriasis Butter – Jar

6 drops Palmarosa
4 drops Patchouli
4 drops Lavender
4 drops Melaleuca Alternifolia
3 drops Roman Chamomile
½ C Coconut Oil
Heat coconut oil in a double boiler until melted. Remove from heat, cool slightly and add essential oils, mixing well. Place bowl in the refrigerator and let cool for approximately 30-60 minutes, until firm but not hardened. Whip with electric mixer until light and airy. Scoop into 4 oz jars. Makes approximately 8 oz.

Scar Prevention – RB

6 drops Myrrh
6 drops Lavender
4 drops Helichrysum
4 drops Sandalwood
Emu Oil
Castor Oil
Top with ½ emu oil and ½ castor oil. Apply to potential scars and massage in as needed.

Scar Remedy – RB

6 drops Helichrysum
4 drops Myrrh
4 drops Lavender
4 drops Sandalwood
2 drops Geranium
Top with Castor Oil. Apply sparingly but frequently on a daily basis to healed scars and massage.

Skin Tags and Warts – Single Application

Oregano
Cotton Swab with CO
Using a toothpick, apply a small amount of Oregano on skin tag or wart. (Helpful hint: This is a hot oil and could burn the skin around it. You may need to use CO on a cotton swab and wipe the skin around the skin tag or wart to protect the surrounding skin before applying the Oregano.) Usually take 1-4 weeks to fall off completely.

Stubborn Warts – Dropper Bottle

3 drops Idaho Balsam Fir
3 drops Lemongrass
3 drops Peppermint
3 drops Lemon
3 drops Frankincense
3 drops Oregano
3 drops Thyme
3 drops Melaleuca Alternifolia
Combine all essential oils in a 10 ml dropper bottle. Top with CO. Apply directly to wart twice daily. Usually takes 1-4 weeks to fall off completely.

Toe Nail Fungus – Dropper Bottle

7 drops Melaleuca Alternifolia
5 drops Oregano
4 drops Thyme
4 drops Lemon
Add all to 2 oz dropper bottle and top with CO. Apply 2-3 times daily. May take 4-6 weeks to see results.

Wellness

Daily Immunity Booster – RB

drops Antibacterial Blend [Recipe on page 19]
3 drops Melaleuca Alternifolia
4 drops Oregano
Top with CO. Apply daily along back of neck, throat, and bottom of feet for added immunity protection.

Weight Loss Trio – Capsules

3 drops Lemon
drops Peppermint
drops Grapefruit
Add essential oils to a size '00' empty vegetable capsule, top with CO and take orally. Also, add a drop of Grapefruit to your water and sip throughout the day to help support flushing the body. Helpful hint: Peppermint, as a natural stimulant, may interrupt your ability to fall asleep. Do not take the capsule too late in the day.)

Advanced Weight Loss – Capsules

drops Lemon (detox)
drops Peppermint (flush)
drops Grapefruit (metabolism)

2 drops Cinnamon Bark (metabolism)

2 drops Ocotea (blood sugar)

Add essential oils to a size '00' empty vegetable capsule, top with CO and take orally. Also, add a drop of Grapefruit to your water and sip throughout the day to help support flushing the body. (Helpful hint: Peppermint, as a natural stimulant, may interrupt your ability to fall asleep. Do not take the capsule too late in the day.)

Meditational Blend Version #1 – Diffuser

4 Frankincense

3 Bergamot

Meditational Blend Version #2 – Diffuser

2 drops Sandalwood

2 drops Frankincense

2 drops Bergamot

Spiritual Grounding Blend - Diffuser

3 drops Cedarwood

3 drops Lavender

2 drops Patchouli

Detox Bath Salts Version #1 – Jar

6 drops Juniper

4 drops Cypress

4 drops Lemongrass

4 drops Lemon

1 C Epsom Salt

1 C Dead Sea Salt (can use additional Epsom Salt if you do not have Dead Sea Salt)

1 C Baking Soda

In a large bowl, thoroughly combine Epsom salt, dead sea salt and baking soda. Add essential oils and stir well. Pour into a 24 oz glass jar. Add 1 cup to running bath water using the hottest tolerable water temperature. Soak 20-30 minutes. Makes enough for 3 baths.

Detox Bath Salts Version #2 – Jar

8 drops Frankincense

7 drops Lavender or Geranium

2 C Epsom Salt

¾ C Baking Soda

¼ C Bentonite Clay

In a large bowl, thoroughly combine Epsom salt, baking soda and bentonite clay. Add essential oils and stir well. Pour into a 24 oz glass jar. Add 1 cup to running bath water using the hottest tolerable water temperature. Soak 20-30 minutes. Makes enough for 3 baths.

Anxiety and Mood Enhancement

Stress and Anxiety Regimen

Diffuse and apply a few drops of Frankincense and Lavender together

Diffuse 4 drops of Spearmint or Orange for a pick-me-up

Apply a few drops of Bergamot, Geranium, Jasmine or Rose over the heart and wrists; Lavender on the back of neck; and a drop or two of Frankincense, Roman Chamomile or Sandalwood on pressure points.

Anti-anxiety – RB

5 drops Lavender
4 drops Vetiver
4 drops Orange
3 drops Frankincense
3 drops Rosewood
3 drops Copaiba
Top with CO. Apply on wrists, back of neck or temples to help ease anxiety.

Panic Go Down – RB

6 drops Vetiver
6 drops Roman Chamomile
4 drops Cedarwood
4 drops Copaiba
2 drops Patchouli
Top with CO. Apply on wrists, back of neck or temples to help promote a sense of peace and calm.

Liquid Calm – RB

drops Copaiba
drops Tangerine
drops Vetiver
drops Patchouli
drops Hong Kuai
drops Blue Tansy
Top with CO. Apply on wrists, back of neck or temples to help promote a sense of peace and calm.

Mellow Momma – RB

drops Lavender
drops Roman Chamomile
drops Clary Sage
drops Vetiver
Top with CO. Apply on wrists, back of neck, temples and bottom of feet to help promote a sense of peace and calm.

Mellow Mix – RB

6 drops Copaiba
5 drops Lavender
4 drops Patchouli
4 drops Vetiver
3 drops Blue Tansy
Top with CO. Apply on wrists, back of neck, temples and bottom of feet as needed for easing anxiety, ADD and ADHD.

Mellow Out – Diffuser

4 drops Manuka
4 drops Grapefruit

Stress Relief! Version #1 – Diffuser

3 drops Grapefruit
1 drop Jasmine
1 drop Ylang Ylang

Stress Relief! Version #2 – Diffuser

4 drops Lavender
2 drops Cedarwood
2 drops Orange
1 drop Ylang Ylang
Optional: 1 drop Vetiver

Stress Reduction Bath Salts Version #1 – Jar

6 drops Bergamot
4 drops Geranium
3 drops Lavender
3 drops Copaiba
1 C Epsom Salt
1 C Baking Soda
½ C Dead Sea Salt (can use additional Epsom Salt if you do not have Dead Sea Salt)
½ C Kosher Salt
In a large bowl, thoroughly combine Epsom salt and baking soda. Add essential oils and stir well. Pour into a 24 oz glass jar. Add 1 cup to running bath water using the hottest tolerable water temperature. Soak 20-30 minutes. Makes enough for 3 baths.

Stress Reduction Bath Salts Version #2 – Jar

7 drops Copaiba
6 drops Cedarwood
5 drops Lime
1 C Epsom Salt

1 C Baking Soda
½ C Dead Sea Salt (can use additional Epsom Salt if you do not have Dead Sea Salt)
½ C Kosher Salt
In a large bowl, thoroughly combine Epsom salt and baking soda. Add essential oils and stir well. Pour into a 24 oz glass jar. Add 1 cup to running bath water using the hottest tolerable water temperature. Soak 20-30 minutes. Makes enough for 3 baths.

Mood Lifting Perfume – RB

5 drops Tangerine
4 drops Clary Sage
3 drops Ylang Ylang
2 drops Lavender
2 drops Bergamot
Top with CO and apply like perfume. This is also good for PMS symptoms.

Happiness Roll On: Version #1 – RB

5 drops Bergamot
4 drops Ylang Ylang
4 drops Ginger
3 drops Geranium
2 drops Cinnamon Bark
Top with CO. Apply to wrists, back of neck, bottom of feet and along collar bone for a pick-me-up.

Happiness Roll On: Version #2 – RB

5 drops Orange
4 drops Frankincense
4 drops Geranium
3 drops Lavender
1 drop Lemon
Top with CO. Apply as needed to wrists, back of neck, bottom of feet and along collar bone for a pick-me-up.

Happiness Roll On: Version 3 – RB

6 drops Lavender
drops Bergamot
drops Frankincense
drops Blue Tansy
drops Lemon
Optional: 3 drops Idaho Blue Spruce
Top with CO. Apply to wrists, back of neck, bottom of feet and along collar bone for a pick-me-up.

Smile Today – RB

drops Lavender

4 drops Vetiver
4 drops Cedarwood
4 drops Marjoram
2 drops Bergamot
Top with CO. Apply on wrists, back of neck or temples to help promote a sense of peace and calm.

Lift Your Mood Version #1 – Diffuser

3 drops Bergamot
3 drops Lavender
2 drops Geranium

Lift Your Mood Version #2 – Diffuser

2 drops Frankincense
1 drop Rose
1 drop Sandalwood

Lift Your Mood Version #3 – Diffuser

4 drops Melissa

Lift Your Mood Version #4 – Diffuser

2 drops Orange
2 drops Bergamot
2 drops Cypress
2 drops Frankincense

Lift Your Mood Version #5 – Diffuser

4 drops Orange
3 drops Peppermint
2 drops Clove

Lift Your Mood Version #6 – Diffuser

4 drops Juniper
3 drops Bergamot

Energize! Recipe #1 – Diffuser

3 drops Grapefruit
2 drops Lavender
2 drops Lemon
1 drop Basil

Energize! Recipe #2 – Diffuser

3 drops Peppermint
3 drops Grapefruit

Optional: 1 drop Rosemary and 2 drops Bergamot for improved focus, energy and alertness.

Energize! Recipe #3 – Diffuser

3 drops Bergamot
3 drops Grapefruit
1 drop Wintergreen

Concentration

Clarifying Study Blend – RB

5 drops Rosemary
5 drops Bergamot
5 drops Basil
3 drops Lemon
3 drops Cypress

Top with CO. Place 1 or 2 drops of the mixture on your fingertips and gently massage your temples. Cup your hands with RB around your nose and mouth and slowly inhale, using the belly breathing technique. Try brief inhalations of the blend while committing facts and figures to memory, and again while trying to recall the information.

Focusing Temple Massage – RB

9 drops Clary Sage
9 drops Bergamot

Top with CO. Use this massage blend to facilitate creative work and to enhance concentration. Place 1 or 2 drops of the mixture on your fingertips and gently massage your temples. Close your eyes as the warm, sweet aroma of the blend penetrates - envision the creative work before you!

Focus Roller – RB

9 drops Frankincense
9 drops Vetiver
4 drops Cedarwood
drops Lavender
drops Basil

Combine all essential oils in a RB, and top with CO. Apply to back of neck, temples, and big toes to promote feelings of concentration.

Mental Clarity Recipe #1 – Diffuser

drops Sandalwood
drops Cedarwood

Mental Clarity Recipe #2 – Diffuser

drops Frankincense

2 drops Vetiver
2 drops Blue Cypress

Mental Clarity Recipe #3 – Diffuser

4 drops Orange
2 drops Peppermint

Stimulant Blend – RB

5 drops Eucalyptus
4 drops Nutmeg
4 drops Lemon
3 drops Black Pepper
2 drops Cinnamon Bark
2 drops Peppermint
Top with CO. Apply along back of neck, temples, wrists and bottom of feet for added energy.

ADD and ADHD Blend #1 – RB

7 drops Lavender
7 drops Cedarwood
7 drops Vetiver
Top with CO. Apply along back of neck, temples, wrists and bottom of feet twice daily.

ADD and ADHD Blend #2 – RB

5 drops Cedarwood
5 drops Frankincense
4 drops Basil
3 drops Lavender
3 drops Patchouli
Top with CO. Apply along back of neck, temples, wrists and bottom of feet twice daily.

ADD and ADHD Blend #3 – RB

6 drops Lavender
5 drops Patchouli
5 drops Cedarwood
4 drops Copaiba
2 drops Rosemary
2 drops Blue Tansy
Top with CO. Apply along back of neck, temples, wrists and bottom of feet twice daily.

Sleep

Relaxation – RB

10 drops Lavender
5 drops Vetiver
4 drops Frankincense
3 drops Orange
Top with CO. Apply as needed to wrists, back of neck and bottom of feet to aid in relaxation.

Relaxation Bath Salts – Jar

15 drops Lavender
2 C Epsom Salt
1 C Baking Soda
In a large bowl, thoroughly combine Epsom salt and baking soda. Add essential oils and stir well. Pour into a 24 oz glass jar. Add 1 cup to running bath water using the hottest tolerable water temperature. Soak 20-30 minutes. Makes enough for 3 baths.

Sleepy Time: Version #1 – RB

5 drops Tangerine
4 drops Ylang Ylang
4 drops Lavender
4 drops Cedarwood
2 drops Sandalwood
2 drops Idaho Balsam Fir
Top with CO. Apply as needed to wrists, back of neck and bottom of feet as an aid for sleep.

Sleepy Time: Version #2 – RB

7 drops Roman Chamomile
5 drops Cedarwood
5 drops Marjoram
drops Lavender
Top with CO. Apply as needed to wrists, back of neck and bottom of feet as an aid for sleep.

Sleepy Time Version #3 – RB

drops Lavender
drops Orange
drops Vetiver
Top with CO. Apply as needed to wrists, back of neck and bottom of feet as an aid for sleep.

Sleepy Time Version #4 – RB

10 drops Roman Chamomile
drops Clary Sage

6 drops Bergamot
Top with CO. Apply as needed to wrists, back of neck and bottom of feet as an aid for sleep.

Sleep Dreams Blend Strong Recipe – RB

6 drops Lavender
5 drops Vetiver
4 drops Valerian
4 drops Cedarwood
4 drops Tangerine
3 drops Juniper
2 drops Clary Sage
2 drops Sandalwood
2 drops Black Spruce
Optional: 2 drops Jasmine
Top with CO. Apply as needed to wrists, back of neck and bottom of feet as an aid for sleep.

Sweet Dreams Bedtime Cream – Jar

10 drops Lavender
10 drops Cedarwood
10 drops Marjoram
8 drops Roman Chamomile
½ C Coconut Oil
Using an electric mixer, whip ingredients until light and airy. Store in an 8 oz glass jar. Rub on bottom of feet at bedtime.

Sleepy – Spray

10 drops Lavender
2 T Witch Hazel
8 T Distilled Water
Add witch hazel and Lavender in a 4 oz spray bottle. Top with distilled water. Shake well before use. Spray on pillows and sheets just before bed.

Sweet Dreams Version #1 – Diffuser

2 drops Lavender
2 drops Marjoram
2 drops Cedarwood

Sweet Dreams Version #2 – Diffuser

3 drops Clary Sage
3 drops Lavender
2 drops Roman Chamomile

Sweet Dreams Version #3 – Diffuser

4 drops Vetiver
2 drops Roman Chamomile
2 drops Valerian

Sweet Dreams Version #4 – Diffuser

4 drops Frankincense
3 drops Lavender
2 drops Mastrante

Sweet Dreams Version #5 – Diffuser

2 drops Bergamot
2 drops Patchouli
2 drops Lavender
2 drops YlangYlang

Bedroom

Libido User Guide

Ylang Ylang: Enhances sensuality, increases libido
Clary Sage: Hormone balancer
Patchouli: Anxiety, decreases inhibitions
Geranium: Hormone balancer, increase libido
Sandalwood: Calming, increase libido
Jasmine: Calming
Lavender: Hormone balancer and increases blood flow and female sensitivity
Clove, Nutmeg, Ginger and Black Pepper: Warming agents
Bergamot: Tension and anxiety
Orange: Emotional Support
Juniper: Evokes feelings of love and peace

Simple Aphrodisiac Blend – Neat

2 drops Bergamot
2 drops Lavender
Diffuse and/or apply neat to reflex points on feet and inner ankles.

Simple Libido Blend – Neat

2 drops Orange
2 drops Rose or Geranium
Diffuse and/or apply neat to reflex points on feet and inner ankles.

In the Mood Version #1 – Diffuser

4 drops Juniper
3 drops Bergamot
1 drop Cinnamon Bark

In the Mood Version #2 – Diffuser

3 drops Lemon Myrtle
2 drops Idaho Blue Spruce
2 drops Nutmeg

In the Mood Version #3 – Diffuser

2 drops Black Spruce
2 drops Ylang Ylang
2 drops Sandalwood
1 drop Geranium

In the Mood Version #4 – Diffuser

3 drops Clary Sage
3 drops Orange
1 drop Jasmine or Rose

Lubricant Recipe – Dropper Bottle

10 drops Ylang Ylang
8 drops Orange
4 drops Lavender
4 drops Geranium
2 drops Peppermint
Optional: 2 drops Melaleuca Alternifolia to stop yeast
Top with fractionated coconut oil in a 1 oz glass dropper bottle and use as needed. (Helpful hint: do not use coconut oil or essential oils with condoms, as they may deteriorate the latex.)

Ready for Love: Hers, Version #1 – Dropper Bottle

10 drops Orange
8 drops Ylang Ylang
6 drops Black Pepper
4 drops Rosewood
2 drops Jasmine
Top with fractionated coconut oil in a 1 oz glass dropper bottle. Apply to inner thighs, lower abdomen, and vita flex points, including inner ankles, 20 minutes before intimacy.

Ready for Love: Hers, Version #2 – Dropper Bottle

10 drops Cary Sage

6 drops Geranium

6 drops Lavender

5 drops Clove

3 drops Peppermint

Top with fractionated coconut oil in a 1 oz glass dropper bottle. Apply to inner thighs, lower abdomen, and vita flex points, including inner ankles, 20 minutes before intimacy.

Ready for Love: His, Version #1 – Dropper Bottle

10 drops Idaho Blue Spruce

5 drops Orange

5 drops Black Pepper

5 drops Ylang Ylang

2 drops Nutmeg

Top with fractionated coconut oil in a 1 oz glass dropper bottle. Apply to inner thighs, lower abdomen, and vita flex points, including inner ankles, 20 minutes before intimacy.

Ready for Love: His, Version #2 – Dropper Bottle

10 drops Idaho Blue Spruce

5 drops Sandalwood

5 drops Cypress

3 drops Nutmeg

Top with fractionated coconut oil in a 1 oz glass dropper bottle. Apply to inner thighs, lower abdomen, and vita flex points, including inner ankles, 20 minutes before intimacy.

Health & Beauty, Face

Face Wash – Foaming Soap Pump Bottle

5 drops Ylang Ylang

7 drops Patchouli

7 drops Frankincense

drops Lemongrass

⅓ C Castile Soap

t Sweet Almond Oil

Optional: 10 drops Sandalwood to assist with wrinkles

Combine all in 8 oz foaming soap pump bottle. Top with distilled water and mix thoroughly. Use twice daily and shake well before use.

Acne Prone Face Wash – Foaming Soap Pump Bottle

drops Patchouli

drops Oregano

drops Melaleuca Alternifolia

drops Lemongrass

4 drops Palmarosa
3 drops Manuka
⅔ C Castile Soap
1 t Sunflower Oil
Combine all in 8 oz foaming soap pump bottle. Top with distilled water and mix thoroughly. Use twice daily and shake well before use.

Face Toner – Spray

4 drops Lavender
4 drops Roman Chamomile
2 drops Frankincense
2 drops Geranium
4 T Alcohol Free Witch Hazel
½ t Sea Salt
Optional: 3 drops Argan Oil
Combine essential oils and sea salt in a 2 oz spray bottle, swirling to mix. Top with Witch Hazel. Use daily after washing face, shake well before use.

Acne Prone Face Toner – Spray

4 drops Lavender
4 drops Melaleuca Alternifolia
2 drops Geranium
2 drops Cypress
4 T Alcohol Free Witch Hazel
½ t Sea Salt
Optional: 3 drops Sunflower Oil
Combine essential oils and sea salt in a 2 oz spray bottle, swirling to mix. Top with witch hazel. Use daily after washing face, shake well before use.

Blemish Gel – Dropper Bottle

10 drops Geranium
10 drops Lavender
6 drops Lemongrass
6 drops Melaleuca Alternifolia.
¼ C Aloe Vera gel
Mix all ingredients and store in 2 oz dropper bottle. Use daily after washing face and applying toner while breakouts are present. Shake well before use.

Daytime Face Serum Version #1 – Dropper Bottle

15 drops Lavender
15 drops Frankincense
2½ T Castor Oil
1½ T Jojoba

Optional: 8 drops Sandalwood to combat an abundance of wrinkles
Combine essential oils in a 2 oz dropper bottle and top with castor oil and jojoba. Use daily after washing face. Shake well before use.

Daytime Face Serum Version #2 – Dropper Bottle

5 drops Frankincense
5 drops Lavender
5 drops Geranium
5 drops Mastrante
3 drops Lemongrass
3 drops Rosemary
2 ½ T Castor Oil
1 ½ T Jojoba
Optional: 8 drops Sandalwood to combat an abundance of wrinkles
Combine essential oils in a 2 oz dropper bottle and top with castor oil and jojoba. Use daily after washing face. Shake well before use.

Face Serum for Combination Skin, Acne and Scarring – Dropper Bottle

10 drops Frankincense
10 drops Lavender
5 drops Palmarosa
5 drops Manuka
Combine essential oils in a 2 oz dropper bottle and top with castor oil and jojoba. Use daily after washing face. Shake well before use.

Lightweight Serum for Large Pores – Dropper Bottle

10 drops Lavender
10 drops Rosemary
10 drops Frankincense
T Argan Oil
T Jojoba
Combine essential oils in 2 oz dropper bottle. Top with argan oil and jojoba, or CO of choice. Use twice daily after washing face until desired results are obtained. Shake well before use.

Moisturizing Nighttime Beauty Serum – Dropper Bottle

drops Geranium
drops Frankincense
drops Lavender
drops Palmarosa
drops Lemon
T Sweet Almond Oil
T Castor Oil
T Vitamin E Oil

Contents of 1 Evening Primrose Capsule

Combine all in 2 oz dropper bottle. Shake gently to mix completely. Use one full dropper every night after washing face.

Moisturizing Nighttime Beauty Serum, Acne Prone – Dropper Bottle

7 drops Lemon

7 drops Lavender

6 drops Palmarosa

5 drops Roman Chamomile

5 drops Frankincense

1 T Argan Oil

1 T Jojoba

Combine essential oils in 2 oz dropper bottle. Top with CO and shake gently to mix completely. Use one full dropper every night after washing face.

The Ultimate Anti-Wrinkle Essential Oil Recipe – Dropper Bottle

5 drops Carrot Seed

5 drops Geranium

5 drops Sandalwood

3 drops Lavender

3 drops Frankincense

3 drops Lemon

3 drops Rosemary

3 drops Patchouli

Argan, Walnut, Sunflower, Jojoba or other CO of choice

Combine all in 2 oz dropper bottle. Top with CO. Shake gently to mix completely. Use one full dropper every night after washing face.

Simple Facial Moisturizing Cream – Jar

12 drops Frankincense

12 drops Lavender

½ C Coconut Oil

Whip coconut oil in a mixer for approximately 5-10 minutes until whipped to a light fluff. Add essential oils above, or your favorite essential oils that are good for skin. Mix well and store in an 8 o[z] glass jar. (Helpful hint: Bear in mind that coconut oil melts at 76°F, so store it in a cool place so it doesn't liquify.)

Blemish Scarring Cream – Jar

12 drops Frankincense

12 drops Lavender

10 drops Helichrysum

10 drops Palmarosa

5 drops Melaleuca Alternifolia

4 T Shea Butter or Coconut Oil

4 T Jojoba or Sunflower Oil

Heat shea butter or coconut oil in a double boiler until melted. Remove from heat and add jojoba or sunflower oil and essential oils, mixing well. Place bowl in the refrigerator and let cool for approximately 30-60 minutes, until firm but not hardened. Whip with electric mixer until light and airy. Scoop into 4 oz jars. Makes approximately 8 oz.

Nighttime Facial Moisturizing Cream – Jar

5 drops Frankincense

5 drops Lavender

5 drops Mastrante

5 drops Lemon

5 drops Geranium

5 drops Lemongrass

1 C Shea Butter

1 C Coconut Oil

2 T Sunflower Oil

2 T Castor Oil

Optional: 5 drops Sandalwood to combat an abundance of wrinkles

Heat shea butter and coconut oil in a double boiler until melted. Remove from heat and add sunflower, castor and essential oils, mixing well. Place bowl in the refrigerator and let cool for approximately 30-60 minutes, until firm but not hardened. Whip with electric mixer until light and airy. Pour in jars. Makes approximately 24 oz. (Note: this is a heavy moisturizer and makes for a somewhat "greasy" feel when you apply this to your skin at night, but know that your skin will adjust to the feeling after a few weeks, and you will see amazing results after regular usage!)

Walnut Eye Cream – Jar

4 drops Frankincense

4 drops Ylang Ylang

4 drops Patchouli

4 drops Lavender

2 T Coconut Oil

1 T Walnut Oil

1 T Grated Beeswax

1 T Rosewater or Distilled Water

Mix together beeswax, coconut and walnut oil in a double boiler and heat gently until the wax is melted. Stirring well, slowly add in the rosewater. Allow the mixture to cool and continue to stir so that the oil and water blend remain mixed. Spoon the cream into a 3 oz glass container. After it cools a bit, stir in the essential oils. This is best used at night, as it is a bit oily.

Facial Sugar Scrub – Jar

10 drops Essential Oil of choice

½ C Granulated or Brown Sugar

Coconut Oil, Olive Oil, Grapeseed, or Sweet Almond Oil

Put sugar in a 4 oz glass jar. Gradually stir in CO until you reach the desired consistency of your scrub, then add in your favorite essential oil(s), stirring well.

Microdermabrasion Scrub – Jar

8 drops Lavender
8 drops Frankincense
6 drops Lemongrass
4 drops Rosemary
5½ T of Baking Soda
2½ T Coconut Oil
6 t Water

Add all ingredients to a glass bowl and thoroughly combine with a fork until well blended. Transfer the scrub to a 4 oz glass jar. To use, apply to a clean face scrubbing lightly in a circular motion. Rinse well, and follow with toner and moisturizer.

Deep Cleansing Clay Mask – Single Application

2 drops Grapefruit
1 drop Geranium
1 drop Juniper
2 T Green Clay
1 t Vegetable Glycerin
3 T Distilled Water

Combine the clay and the floral or distilled water in a bowl and combine well until a thick paste is formed. Add the remaining ingredients and mix well. Spread the mixture over a clean, damp face and neck, avoiding the eye area. Relax for 15 minutes, preferably lying down. Rinse well with warm water before applying a toner and moisturizer. This clay mask recipe is most suitable for oily skin.

Soothing Clay Mask – Single Application

2 drops Roman Chamomile
2 drops Rose
3 T Rose Water or Distilled Water
2 T Red or White Clay
1 t Jojoba

Combine the clay and the floral or distilled water in a bowl and combine well until a thick paste is formed. Add the remaining ingredients and mix well. Spread the mixture over a clean, damp face and neck, avoiding the eye area. Relax for 15 minutes, preferably lying down. Rinse well with warm water before applying a toner and moisturizer. This clay mask recipe is most suitable for dry and sensitive skin. If the facial clay mask dries out too much while applied, you can spritz your face with distilled or floral water.

Revitalizing Clay Mask – Single Application

2 drops Orange
2 drops Petitgrain
1 drop Neroli

2 T Pink Clay

3 T Orange Flower Water or Distilled Water

1 t Vegetable Glycerin

Combine the clay and the flower or distilled water in a bowl and combine well until a thick paste is formed. Add the remaining ingredients and mix well. Spread the mixture over a clean, damp face and neck, avoiding the eye area. Relax for 15 minutes, preferably lying down. Rinse well with warm water before applying a toner and moisturizer. This clay mask recipe is most suitable for dull and tired skins in need of a boost to reclaim that healthy glow.

Facial Clay Mask for Acne – Single Application

2 drops Lavender

1 drop Orange

1 drop Melaleuca Alternifolia

2 T Green Clay

3 T Aloe Vera Gel

1 t Orange Flower Water, Rose Water or Distilled Water

Combine the clay and aloe vera gel in a bowl and combine well. Next, add the flower or distilled water, stirring slowly until a thick paste is formed. Finally, add essential oils and mix well. Spread the mixture over a clean, damp face and neck, avoiding the eye area. Relax for 15 minutes, preferably lying down. Rinse well with warm water before applying a toner and moisturizer. This clay mask recipe is most suitable for acne prone skin.

Glam Glow Face Mask – Single Application

drops Peppermint

drops Eucalyptus

drops Lemon

drops Melaleuca Alternifolia

¼ C Bentonite Clay

T Coconut Oil

capsules of Activated Charcoal

T Aloe Vera Gel

Chamomile Tea Bag

Steep 1 Chamomile tea bag in 4 oz of hot water for approximately 5 minutes. Melt coconut oil in a glass bowl and combine all ingredients except the tea, whisking together well. Slowly begin to add the cooled tea and continue to whisk until a creamy texture is reached. Place the container in the refrigerator for approximately an hour. Spread the mixture over a clean, damp face and neck, avoiding the eye area. Relax for 15 minutes, preferably lying down. Rinse well with warm water before applying a toner and moisturizer. (Helpful hint: You can find activated charcoal in most stores in the vitamin section. Cut the capsules in half and dump the charcoal powder into the bowl to use.)

Homemade Eye Makeup Remover – Jar

drops Lavender

T Coconut Oil

Put the coconut oil in a 1 oz jar, and slowly add the Lavender, mixing thoroughly. To use, simply dip your clean fingertip in the jar and rub over closed eyes on eyelashes to remove mascara.

Lash-Ness

Put 1 drop of Lavender in your existing mascara tube and apply daily as normal for longer, thicker lashes. Alternative: fill a clean, empty mascara tube with enough extra virgin olive oil to come above the brush, and add 3 drops of Lavender. Apply once or twice a day, shaking well before use.

Dark Circles Under Eyes – RB

7 drops Frankincense
7 drops Lavender
7 drops Lemon
Top with CO and roll under eyes twice a day.

Better Bees Lip Balm Base – Lip Balm Tubes

30 drops Essential Oil(s) of choice
2 T Coconut Oil
2 T Beeswax
2 T Shea Butter
17 empty 5.5 ml Lip Balm Tubes

Melt coconut oil, beeswax, and shea butter in a double boiler. Remove from heat, add essential oils and stir. Use a pipette to fill empty lip balm tubes or small salve jars. Let the lip balm tubes sit for about 30 minutes to harden. Makes approximately 17 5.5 ml tubes.

- Helpful hint #1: During winter months, reduce the amount of beeswax to 1 tablespoon to prevent over-hardening.
- Helpful hint #2: After melting, you can add 1 tablespoon of vitamin e oil and 1 tablespoon of sweet almond oil for additional softness, or ¼ of a teaspoon of honey and ¼ of a teaspoon of vanilla extract for a slightly different flavor.
- Helpful hint #3: Essential oils that are good for lip care include German Chamomile, Geranium, Lavender, Frankincense, Jasmine, Lemon and Melaleuca Alternifolia.
- Helpful hint #4: Possible ideas for creative combinations include Lavender/Peppermint, Lemon/Lime, Lavender/Lemon, Spearmint/Grapefruit, Cinnamon Bark/Lemon, Melaleuca Alternifolia/Grapefruit, Melaleuca Alternifolia/Rosemary, Clove/Orange… Possibilities are endless, don't be afraid to experiment!

Cinnamon Bark and Orange Lip Balm – Tubes

15 drops Cinnamon Bark
10 drops Orange
1 ½ T Beeswax Pellets
1 T Coconut Oil
1 T Shea Butter
2 T Sweet Almond Oil
13 empty 5.5 ml Lip Balm Tubes

Place beeswax, coconut oil and shea butter in a double boiler over low heat. Stir until completely melted and remove from heat. Add sweet almond oil and essential oils, stirring well. Use a pipette to fill empty lip balm tubes or small salve jars. Let the lip balm tubes sit for about 30 minutes to harden. Makes approximately 13 tubes. This recipe is great during cooler months!

Lip Scrub – Jar

3 drops Lavender
3 drops Lemon
3 T Cane or Coconut Sugar
1 T Jojoba
1 ½ t Honey
1 drop Vitamin E Oil

In a 2 oz glass jar, mix jojoba, vitamin e oil and honey until thoroughly combined. Add essential oils. Slowly mix in sugar until you reach your desired consistency.

Lip Plumper

5 drops Peppermint
1 T Coconut Oil
¼ t Jojoba
¼ t Sweet Almond Oil

Combine all in a small container and apply to lips for a natural tingling/plumping effect.

Health & Beauty, Hair

Hair Regrowth Shampoo and Conditioner – Additive

-2 drops per oz Cedarwood
-2 drops per oz Lavender
-2 drops per oz Rosemary
-2 drops per oz Thyme

Add the above essential oils to your favorite shampoo and conditioner. Mix thoroughly, and shake well before use.

Hair Regrowth – Spray

drops Cedarwood
drops Lavender
drops Rosemary
drops Thyme
T Alcohol-Free Witch Hazel
Distilled Water

Add all ingredients to a 4 oz glass spray bottle and top with distilled water. Spritz on scalp daily, combing through at the roots. Use this in conjunction with the Hair Regrowth Shampoo and Conditioner Additive recipe, as well as the Hair Regrowth Masque.

Hair Regrowth Masque – Dropper Bottle

8 drops Cedarwood
8 drops Lavender
8 drops Rosemary
8 drops Thyme
4 T Pure, Refined Organic Emu Oil
4 T Jojoba

Combine essential oils and emu oil in a 4 oz glass dropper bottle. Top with jojoba, argan, tamanu or other CO of choice. To use, apply to clean, damp hair and leave on overnight or for 12 hours. Use 2-3 times weekly.

Rosemary Peppermint Shampoo – Bottle

12 drops Rosemary
4 drops Peppermint
1½ C Castile Soap
½ C Distilled Water
1 t Argan Oil
1 t Vegetable Glycerin

Add castile soap to a 16 oz container with a flip top lid. Next, add argan oil, vegetable glycerin and essential oils. Top with ½ cup distilled water. Shake well before use. Use as you would any shampoo, but have the expectation of minimal lather.

Lavender and Rosemary Shampoo – Bottle

10 drops Lavender
6 drops Rosemary
4 drops Ylang Ylang
1½ C Castile Soap
½ C Distilled Water
1 T Jojoba
1 t Vegetable Glycerin

Add castile soap to a 16 oz container with a flip top lid. Next, add jojoba, argan oil, vegetable glycerin and essential oils. Top with ½ cup distilled water. Shake well before use. Use as you would any shampoo, but have the expectation of minimal lather.

Rosemary Peppermint Shampoo with Coconut Milk Base – Bottle

12 drops Rosemary
4 drops Peppermint
1⅓ C Coconut Milk
⅔ C Castile Soap
1 t Argan Oil
1 t Vitamin E Oil
1 t Vegetable Glycerin

Add castile soap to a 16 oz container with a flip top lid. Next, add coconut milk, argan oil, vitamin e oil, vegetable glycerin and essential oils. Shake well before use. Use as you would any shampoo, with the expectation of a good amount of lather.

Shampoo Recipe Using Organic Base – Bottle

15 drops Essential Oil(s) of choice
2 C Organic Shampoo Base (I prefer Stephenson's Brand™)
1 T Coconut Oil
1 t Tamanu Oil (for dry hair or scalp)

Add organic shampoo base to a 16 oz container with a flip top lid. Next, add all other ingredients and combine thoroughly. Shake well before use. Use as you would any shampoo and have the expectation of a good amount of lather. (Helpful Hint: Add essential oils to suit your individual needs. Oils that help with dry scalp include Cedarwood, Lavender, Geranium and Patchouli. Peppermint, Lemon and Lavender aid with an oily scalp, while Melaleuca Alternifolia has been shown to be helpful with dandruff. Clary Sage, Thyme, Roman Chamomile and Lavender help with damaged hair.)

Conditioner Recipe Using Organic Base – Bottle

15 drops Essential Oil(s) of choice
2 C Organic Shampoo Base (I prefer Stephenson's Brand™)
1 T Tamanu Oil (for dry hair or scalp)

Add organic conditioner base to a 16 oz container with a flip top lid. Next, add all other ingredients and mix well. Once the conditioner sets up, after a few hours, you can add a small amount of water if necessary to thin to your preference. Shake well before use. After shampooing hair, condition from root to ends and let sit for 3-5 minutes, rinsing well afterwards.

Deep Treat Hair Conditioner – Jar

10 drops Essential Oil(s) of choice
6 T Coconut Oil
3 T Shea Butter
1 T Argan Oil

Melt coconut oil and shea butter together in a microwave or double boiler, stirring until thoroughly combined. Let mixture cool slightly then add argan oil. Whisk together for 3-5 minutes, then store in a 5 oz glass jar. To use, comb through clean, dry hair and let sit for 30 minutes. Rinse hair and shampoo as normal.

Hair Conditioning Oil – Jar

20 drops Essential Oil(s) of choice
8 T Jojoba or Argan Oil

Mix the jojoba and essential oil(s) in a 4 oz glass jar. Using only your fingertips, dip a few drops of oil onto your hands and lightly run through your hair for added shine. (Helpful hint: Suggestions for this recipe include Rosemary, Basil, Chamomile, Cedarwood, Geranium, Clary Sage, Eucalyptus, Lavender, Lemon, Lemongrass, Patchouli, Peppermint, Myrrh, Sage, Melaleuca Alternifolia, Thyme or Ylang Ylang.)

Dry Shampoo – Shaker Bottle

8 drops Essential Oil(s) of choice
½ C Arrowroot Powder
Optional: 1 T Cocoa Powder for dark hair
Combine all ingredients in a 6 oz shaker bottle, mixing well. Sprinkle in your hair along the roots and style, brushing out excess as you go. You will gain volume and your hair will smell amazing!

Dry Shampoo - Spray

8 drops Essential Oil of choice
1 T Arrowroot Powder
8 T Distilled Water
Optional: 1 t Cocoa Powder for dark hair
Combine all in spray bottle, mixing well. Spray in hair at roots, style, and let air dry.

Hair Detangler Version #1 – Spray

6 drops Lavender
4 drops Orange
2 drops Rosemary
1 T Vegetable Glycerin
¼ t Vitamin E Oil
7 T Aloe Vera
Combine all in 4 oz glass spray bottle. Shake well before use. Apply to damp hair at the roots and brush through to ends.

Hair Detangler Version #2 – Spray

4 drops Orange
3 drops Lavender
3 drops Cedarwood
2 drops Melaleuca Alternifolia
1 T Vegetable Glycerin
¼ t Vitamin E Oil
7 T Aloe Vera
Combine all in 4 oz glass spray bottle. Shake well before use. Apply to damp hair at the roots and brush through to ends.

Beachy Hair Spritz – Spray

10 drops Essential Oil(s) of choice
1 C Hot Water
1 T Sea Salt
2 t Fractionated Coconut Oil
1 t Aloe Vera Gel
Optional - 1 t Epsom Salt for conditioning
Optional - 1 T Sugar for volume and hold

Pour all ingredients, except essential oils, into a 10 oz bottle and shake until dissolved. Add essential oils of choice, and mix well. Shake well before use. To use, spray into damp hair and finger curl into sections, allowing to dry naturally. Or for added boost at roots, spray into damp hair and blow dry. A third option is to spray into dry hair, scrunch and twirl!

Health & Beauty, Body

Peppermint Sugar Scrub Bar – Soap

15 drops Peppermint
1½ C Sugar
1 C Melt and Pour Soap Base, cubed
½ C Sweet Almond Oil
¼ C Unused Coffee Grounds
Silicone Molds
On the stovetop in a double boiler, combine soap base and sweet almond oil, heating until liquefied. Remove from heat and add sugar, coffee grounds and essential oil. Carefully pour contents into silicone molds. Let them cool until firmly set, then store in an airtight container until ready to use.

Cinnamon Bark and Orange Soap – Bars

20 drops Orange
15 drops Cinnamon Bark
10 drops Clove
2 lbs. Clear Organic Glycerin Melt and Pour Soap Base, cubed
Silicone Mold of choice
On the stovetop in a double boiler, heat melt and pour soap base until liquified. Add in essential oils and stir completely. Let your nose be your guide and add additional drops if needed. Pour into molds and let solidify for at least 45 minutes. When completely hardened, remove from molds and store individually wrapped or in an airtight container.

Lemon and Chamomile Bubble Bath – Bottle

10 drops Lemon
10 drops Roman Chamomile
1¼ C Castile Soap
½ C Vegetable Glycerin
¼ C Water
1 t Vitamin E Oil
Mix all ingredients except water in a 16 oz glass bottle. Top with water to desired consistency, mixing thoroughly as you go. Shake well before use.

Lavender and Honey Body Wash – Bottle

20 drops Lavender
1⅓ C Castile Soap
½ C Honey

4 t Vegetable Glycerin
4 t Sweet Almond Oil
2 t Vitamin E Oil
Combine all ingredients in a 16 oz glass bottle. Shake well before use.

Creamy Body Wash Recipe – Bottle

30 drops Essential Oil(s) of choice
2 C Castile Soap
1 C Coconut Oil
1 C Sweet Almond Oil
1 T Vegetable Glycerin
1 t Vitamin E Oil
In a double boiler, slowly melt coconut oil. Once melted, remove from heat, and using an electric mixer, slowly add in all other ingredients and blend thoroughly. Pour into a 32 oz jug. Shake well before use.

Lavender Lemongrass Moisturizer – Spray

5 drops Lavender
5 drops Lemongrass
1½ t Vegetable Glycerin
1 t Sweet Almond Oil
4 drops Vitamin E Oil
⅓ C Distilled Water
Combine all ingredients except water in a 4 oz glass spray bottle. When combined, top with distilled water. Shake well before use. Apply to legs, feet, elbows and hands after showering. No need to rub it in, so it is the perfect time saver.

Shave Cream – Jar

15 drops Essential Oil(s) of choice
½ C Coconut Oil
½ C Shea Butter
½ T Baking Soda
¼ C Avocado or Almond Oil
Mix together coconut oil and shea butter in a double boiler, and heat over low heat. When melted, remove from heat and add ¼ cup avocado or almond oil and 15 drops essential oil(s) of choice. Let sit for 30-45 minutes in the refrigerator, until firm but not hardened. Using an electric mixer, whip for approximately 5-10 minutes, while adding in a ½ tablespoon of baking soda, until mixture is light and airy. Makes approximately 16 oz. Store in airtight glass jars. A little bit goes a long way and after using, you won't need any lotion! Caution: You will need a non-slip bath mat because this can make the bathtub very slick.

Aftershave Cream – Jar

8 drops Lavender
6 drops Roman Chamomile

4 drops Melaleuca Alternifolia
½ C Coconut Oil
½ C Shea Butter
1 T Almond oil

Mix together coconut oil and shea butter in a double boiler, and heat over low heat. When melted, remove from heat and add 1 tablespoon of almond oil and essential oils. Let sit for 30-45 minutes in the refrigerator, until firm but not hardened. Using an electric mixer, whip for approximately 5-10 minutes until mixture is light and airy. Makes approximately 16 oz. Store in airtight glass jars.

Bust Firming Oil – Dropper Bottle

8 drops Lemon
8 drops Geranium
8 drops Orange
8 drops Ylang Ylang
6 drops Lemongrass
5 drops Carrot Seed
4 T Sweet Almond Oil
2 T Extra Virgin Olive Oil
2 T Argan Oil

Mix all ingredients in a 2 oz dropper bottle. Massage into breasts (avoiding the nipples) twice daily to help firm the breasts as well as rejuvenate the skin.

Bath Salts – Jar

15 drops Essential Oil(s) of choice
2 C Epsom Salt
1 C Baking Soda

In a large bowl, thoroughly combine Epsom salt and baking soda. Add essential oils and stir well. Pour into a 24 oz glass jar. Add 1 cup to running bath water using the hottest tolerable water temperature. Soak 20-30 minutes. Makes enough for 3 baths.

Bath Bombs for Humid Climates

20-25 drops Essential Oil(s) of choice
1 C Baking Soda
½ C Epsom Salt
½ C Arrowroot Powder
½ C Citric Acid
¼ t Water
2 t Jojoba or Sweet Almond Oil
Silicone Molds

Preheat oven to 200°F. While oven is preheating, combine baking soda, Epsom salt and arrowroot powder in a bowl. In a separate bowl, combine water, jojoba or sweet almond oil and essential oils. Mix the wet ingredient mixture into the dry ingredient mixture. Using your hands, continue to combine until it's like wet sand. In the beginning it will seem insufficient, but just keep going - It is enough and it WILL take on the correct consistency. After you have wet sand consistency, add citric acid and combine completely. There should be NO fizzing. If you have any fizz, it is too wet. After combined, pack hard into silicone molds, (example: the half sphere 2 3/4" molds). The harder you pack, the less likely to crack! Place your filled molds onto a baking sheet and place in oven. Turn the oven OFF. Let sit in for a few hours, then pop out of molds and lay them flat surface down. Return to oven and let sit overnight. Package and store in airtight container.

Chocolate Ice Cream Bath Truffles

20-30 drops Essential Oil of choice
1¼ C Baking Soda
¾ C Citric Acid
5 T Cocoa Powder
4 T Cocoa Butter
2 T Shea Butter

Melt shea butter and cocoa butter in a double boiler and set aside. When cooled slightly, add essential oil. In a separate mixing bowl, gently sift together dry ingredients. Add melted butters to powdered mixture and mix well. Working quickly, scoop mixture with an ice cream scoop and place on parchment paper. Let dry until firm and store in an airtight container.

Scrubs

Brown Sugar Scrub – Jar

10 drops Lavender OR Essential Oil(s) of choice
1 C White Sugar
1 C Brown Sugar
3 T Olive Oil

Place sugar in a bowl, slowly stirring in the olive oil until desired consistency and texture are reached. Add essential oils, stirring until well blended. Store in two 8 oz glass jars. To use, place a spoonful on skin, scrub gently in a circular motion, and rinse well.

Cinnamon Bark Vanilla Sugar Scrub – Jar

10 drops Cinnamon Bark
2 C Packed Brown Sugar
¼ C Coconut Oil
½ t Vanilla Extract

Place sugar in a bowl, slowly stirring in the coconut oil until desired consistency and texture are reached. Add vanilla extract and Cinnamon Bark, stirring well. Store in two 8 oz glass jars. To use, place a spoonful on skin, scrub gently in a circular motion, and rinse well.

Peppermint Sugar Scrub – Jar

10 drops Peppermint
2 C Turbinado Sugar or Thick Granulated Sugar
¼ C Sweet Almond Oil
Optional: Natural Food Coloring

Place sugar in a bowl, slowly stirring in the almond oil until desired consistency and texture are reached. Add Peppermint, still stirring, and food coloring if desired. Store in two 8 oz glass jars. To use, place a spoonful on skin, scrub gently in a circular motion, and rinse well.

Lavender Lemon Sugar Scrub – Jar

5 drops Lavender
5 drops Lemon
1 C Brown Sugar
¾ C White Sugar
¼ C Coconut Oil

Place sugar in a bowl, slowly pressing in the coconut oil and stirring until desired consistency and texture are reached. Add Lavender and Lemon, stirring until well blended. Store in two 8 oz glass jars. To use, place a spoonful on skin, scrub gently in a circular motion, and rinse well.

Winter Smooth Hand Scrub – Jar

10 drops Lavender or Essential Oil(s) of choice
1 C White Sugar
1 C Brown Sugar
⅔ C Olive Oil
1 t Vitamin E Oil

Place sugar in a bowl, slowly stirring in the olive oil and vitamin e oil until desired consistency and texture are reached. Add Lavender or essential oils of choice, stirring until well blended. Store in two 8 oz glass jars. To use, place a spoonful on skin, scrub gently in a circular motion, and rinse well.

Cellulite Fighting Scrub – Jar

10 drops Grapefruit
10 drops Tangerine
2 C White Sugar
½ C Coconut Oil
1 T Coffee Grounds (unused)

Place sugar in a bowl, slowly stirring in the coconut oil until desired consistency and texture are reached. Add essential oils and coffee grounds, stirring until well blended. Store in two 8 oz glass jars. To use, place a spoonful on skin, scrub gently in a circular motion, and rinse well.

Orange Cream Sugar Scrub – Jar

10 drops Orange
2 C White Sugar
¼ C Coconut Oil
1 t Vanilla Extract

Place sugar in a bowl, slowly stirring in the coconut oil until desired consistency and texture are achieved. Add Orange, stirring until well blended. Store in two 8 oz glass jars. To use, place a spoonful on skin, scrub gently in a circular motion, and rinse well.

Lotions and Creams

Whipped Hand Cream – Jar

15 drops Lavender
10 drops Geranium
5 drops Melaleuca Alternifolia
¼ C Coconut Oil
¼ C Shea Butter
¼ C Cocoa Butter

In a double boiler over medium heat, melt the coconut oil, shea butter and cocoa butter. Stir. Remove from heat and pour in a mixing bowl. Place mixing bowl in refrigerator for about an hour until the mixture is firm but not hardened. Remove from refrigerator and begin mixing in electric mixer on a low speed. Increase the speed of the mixer to high. Add essential oils. Whip mixture for about 10 minutes until light and airy. Makes approximately 12 oz. Spoon body butter into container of choice. (Helpful hint: cocoa butter can be purchased as regular scent, which smells of chocolate, or deodorized, with no smell, depending on your preference.)

Lavender Hand Cream – Jar

20 drops Lavender
½ C Coconut Oil
½ C Olive Oil
¼ C Beeswax Pastilles
½ T Vitamin E Oil

Melt coconut, olive oil and beeswax in a double boiler. When melted, remove from heat, cool slightly and add Lavender and vitamin e oil. Pour into a 10 oz glass jar.

Whipped Lotion Base – Jar

30 drops Essential Oil(s) of choice
1¼ C Shea Butter
½ C Coconut Oil
½ C Sweet Almond Oil

In a double boiler over medium heat, melt coconut oil and shea butter, stirring well. Remove from heat and place in refrigerator for about 30-60 minutes until the mixture is firm but not hardened. Remove from refrigerator and mix on low speed. Add almond oil slowly to the mixture. Gradually increase the speed of the mixer to high. Add essential oils of choice. Whip mixture for approximately 5-10 minutes until light and airy. Spoon into containers. Makes approximately 30 oz, depending on how long you whip it. See the following combination ideas:

Stretch Marks 4 drops Elemi, 4 drops Lemongrass, 4 drops Lavender, 4 drops Frankincense, 4 drops Melaleuca Alternifolia, 4 drops Myrrh, 4 drops Peppermint, 4 drops Basil

Bust Firming Cream 4 drops Vetiver, 4 drops Geranium, 4 drops Ylang Ylang, 4 drops Frankincense, 4 drops Orange, 4 drops Lemongrass, 4 drops Lemon, 4 drops Argan Oil

Dry Skin 6 drops Lavender, 6 drops Geranium, 6 drops Frankincense, 6 drops Myrrh (or Melaleuca Alternifolia)

Eczema **6 drops Helichrysum, 6 drops Lavender, 6 drops Patchouli, 6 drops Melaleuca Alternifolia, 6 drops German Chamomile**

Relaxation **10 drops Mastrante, 6 drops Lavender, 6 drops Bergamot, 4 Clary Sage**

Manly Lime **8 drops Cedarwood, 6 drops Lime, 4 drops Copaiba, 4 drops Lavender,**

Peace **12 drops Bergamot, 8 drops Juniper, 4 drops Marjoram or Lavender**

Basic Body Butters

Whipped Body Butter – Jar

15-20 drops Essential Oil(s) of choice
¾ C Shea Butter
½ C Horsetail Butter
½ C Avocado Oil
¼ C Cocoa Butter
1 t Vitamin E Oil
1 t Corn Starch

Melt cocoa butter, horsetail butter and shea butter in a double boiler slowly. When melted, remove from heat and add avocado oil, vitamin e oil and essential oils. Whisk in corn starch. Put in refrigerator for 30-60 minutes until mixture is firm but not hardened. Remove and use hand or electric mixer to whip for approximately 5-10 minutes. This will make approximately 20 oz.

Listed below are numerous deviations for Whipped Body Butters, all with the same concept: Heat CO's in a double boiler on medium heat, then place the bowl in the refrigerator for approximately 30-60 minutes until the mixture is firm but not hard. Remove from refrigerator and mix with an electric mixer on low speed. Gradually increase speed, add essential oils and whip for approximately 5-10 minutes until light and airy. Most recipes make multiple jars. (Helpful hint: Cocoa Butter can be purchased as regular scent, which smells of chocolate, or deodorized, with no smell.)

Lemon Meringue Body Butter – Jar

16 drops Lemon
1 C Shea Butter
½ C Cocoa Butter
¼ C Hemp Seed Oil
¼ C Avocado oil

Chocolate Spice Body Butter – Jar

10 drops Cinnamon Bark
6 drops Clove
4 drops Nutmeg
1 C Cocoa Butter
⅔ C Shea Butter
⅓ C Sweet Almond Oil

Chocolate Soufflé Body Butter – Jar

15 drops Orange
1 C Shea Butter
½ C Coconut Oil
¼ C Cocoa Powder
2 t Vanilla Extract

Citrus Body Butter – Jar

4 drops Lime
4 drops Lemon
4 drops Orange
4 drops Tangerine
1 C Shea Butter
⅓ C Deodorized Cocoa Butter
⅓ C Avocado Oil

Coconut Lime Butter – Jar

16 drops Lime
1 C Shea Butter
1 C Coconut Oil

Baby Massage Butter – Jar

12 drops Lavender
1 C Shea Butter
½ C Deodorized Cocoa Butter
⅓ C Sweet Almond Oil

Summertime Easy Butter – Jar

14 drops Grapefruit
1 C Cocoa Butter
⅓ C Shea Butter
½ C Coconut Oil
This recipe is firm, so it will be soft in summer months but not too hard to use during winter months.

Pregnant Belly Butter – Jar

8 drops Essential Oil(s) of choice
1¼ C Shea Butter
1 C Sweet Almond Oil
½ C Mango Butter
Leave essential oils out in the first trimester.

Gardening Hand Butter – Jar

16 drops Lavender
⅔ C Olive Oil, infused with 2 T of Lavender buds and 2 T of Chamomile flowers
1⅓ C Shea Butter

Under Eye Butter – Jar

8 drops Carrot Seed
½ C Mango Butter
¼ C Coconut Oil

Silky Body Butters

Orange Ylang Ylang Body Butter – Jar

14 drops Ylang Ylang
7 drops Orange
1 C Shea Butter
½ C Coconut Oil
½ C Cocoa Butter
¼ C Sweet Almond Oil
½ T Vitamin E Oil
1 T Arrowroot Powder

Summertime Butter – Jar

8 drops Lavender
6 drops Orange
4 drops Geranium
1 C Shea Butter
½ C Cocoa Butter
½ C Coconut Oil
2 t Arrowroot Powder

Feet Butter – Jar

18 drops Peppermint
1½ C Shea Butter
½ C Coconut Oil
2 t Arrowroot Powder

Sensitive Skin Butter – Jar

8 drops Neroli
5 drops Lavender
1 C Coconut Oil
½ C Cocoa Butter

1 t Arrowroot Powder

Overnight Butter – Jar

18 drops Lavender
1½ C Shea Butter
¾ C Coconut Oil
2 t Arrowroot Powder

Calming Butter for Kids – Jar

14 drops Lavender
1¼ C Shea Butter
½ C Coconut Oil
2 t Arrowroot Powder

Tropical Herbal Butter – Jar

10 drops Carrot Seed
4 drops Lavender
3 drops Basil
1 C Shea Butter
½ C Coconut Oil
½ C Mango Butter
1 t Vanilla Extract
2 t Arrowroot Powder

Health & Hygiene

Hand Sanitizer – Spray

20 drops Antibacterial Blend [Recipe on page 19]
8 T Alcohol-Free Witch Hazel
2 T Aloe Vera Gel
2 t Vitamin E Oil
1 t Sea Salt
6 T Distilled Water
Add Antibacterial Blend and sea salt into an 8 oz glass spray bottle, swirling to mix. Continue to add all other ingredients except water, mixing as you go. Top with distilled water. Shake well before use.

Hand Sanitizer – Bottle

5 drops Antibacterial Blend [Recipe on page 19]
2 drops Peppermint
1 t Aloe Vera Gel
⅛ t Vitamin E Oil
1 T Distilled Water

Combine the aloe vera gel, vitamin e oil and essential oils into a 2 oz squeeze bottle. Add distilled water to thin the mixture a bit; you'll want it just thin enough to coat your hand.

Sanitizing Hand Soap – Foaming Soap Pump Bottle

12 drops Antibacterial Blend [Recipe on page 19]
10 drops Lemon
10 drops Orange
⅓ C Castile Soap
1 T Aloe Vera Gel
1 T of your preferred brand of All-Natural Household Cleaner
1 t Sweet Almond Oil or Vitamin E Oil
Distilled Water
Combine all ingredients except distilled water in an 8 oz foaming soap pump bottle. Mix well and top with distilled water. Shake well before use.

Liquid Hand Soap – Foaming Soap Pump Bottle

10-15 drops Peppermint or Essential Oil of choice
⅓ C Castile Soap
1 t Vitamin E Oil
⅔ C Distilled Water
Mix soap, vitamin e oil and Peppermint in an 8 oz foaming soap pump bottle. Top with distilled water. Shake well before use.

Toothpaste – Jar

1 drop Melaleuca Alternifolia
1 drop Peppermint (or to taste)
7 T Calcium Magnesium Powder
5 T Coconut Oil
2 T Baking Soda
Mix ingredients well and store in an 8 oz glass jar.

Mouthwash – Bottle

10 drops Antibacterial Blend [Recipe on page 19]
4 drops Peppermint
2 drops Frankincense
2 drops Spearmint
1 t Baking Soda
¼ t Sea Salt
1 C Distilled Water
Combine all ingredients except water in an 8 oz bottle. When mixed well, top with distilled water. Shake well before use. Rinse mouth with 1 tablespoon as needed - Gargle, swish, spit! Though a bit strange to adjust to at first, this mouthwash is very different from most commercial options available which contain alcohol and synthetics. After a few weeks, you will most likely prefer this natural alternative.

Deodorant Detox – Spray

4 drops Rosemary
4 drops Lavender
1 T Apple Cider Vinegar
3 T Distilled Water

Mix all ingredients in a 2 oz glass spray bottle. Shake well before use. Sometimes transitioning to a natural deodorant can create a bit of a "sticky" situation. This simple spray can help detox your armpits and make a successful transition. It can take 2-3 weeks for your body to adjust to an aluminum-free deodorant. Use this spray nightly for 2 weeks. During the first week, refrain from wearing deodorant. During the second week, begin to incorporate your natural deodorant. Continue using for a third week if necessary. Be sure to drink plenty of water to aid in this process!

Deodorant – Jar

10 drops Essential Oil of choice
¼ C Baking Soda
¼ C Arrowroot Powder
6 T Coconut Oil

Mix all ingredients in an 8 oz jar. It will have a consistency like cake icing when finished. Use approximately ½ teaspoon under each arm. (Helpful hint: Lemon, as well as Lemongrass, are popular deodorant preferences for both their aroma and anti-bacterial properties.)

Lavender and Lemongrass Deodorant – Jar

5 drops Lavender
5 drops Lemongrass
3 T Coconut Oil
3 T Baking Soda
2 T Shea Butter
2 T Arrowroot Powder

Melt coconut oil and shea butter in a double boiler over medium heat until melted. Remove from heat and slowly stir in baking soda and arrowroot powder, mixing well. Add essential oils and pour into a 5 oz glass jar for storage. If you prefer, you can pour into a deodorant stick for easier use, though it may melt in the summer.

Deodorant – Spray

30 drops Lemon or Lemongrass
15 drops Lavender
5 drops Melaleuca Alternifolia
¼ C Apple Cider Vinegar
¼ C Distilled Water

Mix all ingredients in a 4 oz glass spray bottle. Shake well before use. (Helpful hint: Cypress, Petitgrain, Sage, Idaho Blue Spruce and Melaleuca Alternifolia make other good deodorant choices.)

Grapefruit Cypress Deodorant – Stick

30 drops Grapefruit
20 drops Cypress
½ C Coconut Oil
½ C Shea Butter
¼ C Cocoa Butter
¼ C Beeswax
6 T Baking Soda
6 T Arrowroot Powder
2 T Bentonite Clay

Melt coconut oil, shea butter, cocoa butter and beeswax in a double boiler over medium heat until melted. Remove from heat and slowly stir in baking soda, bentonite clay and arrowroot powder, mixing well. Add essential oils and pour into empty deodorant containers. Let the deodorant sticks thoroughly dry for 24 hours, and then cap and store. Yields approximately 13 ounces. (Helpful hints: For a firmer stick, add more beeswax. For a softer stick, add more coconut oil. And if you prefer a white deodorant, skip the bentonite clay and add another 2 tablespoons of arrowroot powder. However, bentonite clay has so many amazing healing benefits, I would leave this in the recipe!)

Stinky Piggy Powder – Shaker Bottle

5 drops Peppermint
5 drops Melaleuca Alternifolia
5 drops Sage
⅓ C Cornstarch
⅓ C Baking Soda

Mix all together well in a 6 oz shaker bottle. Sprinkle 1 teaspoon into the heels of both shoes every night, and tip/swish the powder down into the toes of each shoe. In the morning, remove the excess powder.

Stinky Piggy Bath Salts – Jar

12 drops Lemon
8 drops Melaleuca Alternifolia
2 C Baking Soda
1 C Epsom Salt
1 C Dead Sea Salt

In a large bowl, thoroughly combine Epsom salt and dead sea salt. Mix in baking soda and add essential oils, stirring well. Pour into a 24 oz glass jar. For harsh foot odors, use this recipe nightly for a week. Using a bowl large enough to encompass both feet, add the hottest water possible along with a ½ cup of the salts. Soak feet for 15-20 minutes, and during the last few minutes, using a washcloth, scrub feet thoroughly from top to bottom. Makes enough for 6 foot baths.

Sunscreen – Jar

30 drops Carrot Seed (SPF 35-40)
30 drops Red Raspberry Seed Oil (SPF 25-50)

¼ C Coconut Oil (SPF 4)

¼ C Sweet Almond Oil (SPF 5)

3 T Beeswax

2 T Shea Butter (SPF 4-5)

2 T + 2 t Non-Nano Zinc Oxide (SPF 2-20)

½ t Vitamin E Oil

In a double boiler, add all ingredients except zinc oxide, Red Raspberry and Carrot Seed Oils. When melted completely, remove from heat and add zinc oxide SLOWLY (do not inhale the powder, use a mask if needed). Cool slightly, then add Red Raspberry and Carrot Seed Oils. Place in the refrigerator for approximately 30-60 minutes, until firm but not hardened. Using an electric mixer, whip for approximately 5-10 minutes until light and airy. Store in a 6 oz container. This has an SPF around 40, but will vary depending on how much of each product is added. It has the consistency of a buttercream frosting and smells like peach pie. Be sure to reapply every few hours or after being in the water. (Helpful hint: Before placing the mixture in the refrigerator to firm up, grab an empty deodorant tube and fill it up. Let it sit without the top for a few hours to firm. This gives you a handy sunscreen stick that works great on faces, in addition to the sunscreen cream that you will create!)

Inhaler Combinations

Use 12 drops per inhaler total. Sample ideas include:

Fatigue Rosemary, Basil, Peppermint, OR Lavender, Peppermint, Rosemary, Sage

Moody Cedar, Cypress, Lavender, Tangerine

Happy Lemon, Bergamot, Jasmine, Sage

Calming Lemon, Bergamot, Orange

Headache Lavender, Peppermint, Marjoram

Alertness Peppermint, Eucalyptus, Rosemary, Cedarwood, Ravintsara

Stress Lavender, Sandalwood, Patchouli, Bergamot

Studying Rosemary, Clove, Basil, Black Pepper, Helichrysum

Uplifting Grapefruit, Mandarin, Orange, Spearmint

Children

It is IMPERATIVE that you check the safety of essential oils as well as research their properties before applying on children. Some essential oils such as Peppermint are not recommended on children younger than 30 months, and Rosemary should not be used on children younger than 4. It is critical that you do your research and investigate the safety of any essential oil that you plan to use.

It is equally imperative that you check all dilution requirements and recommendations. Individual dilution ratios can be found on quality essential oil bottles. Essential oils applied topically to children must be at minimum diluted further than the label states. For example: Thyme requires a dilution rate of 1:4, which equals 1 drop Thyme and 4 drops CO for adults. You then further dilute by age using the recommended dilution chart for children below. For a child ages 6 months-2 years, it would be 4x label recommendations, which is 1:16 (1 drop EO:16 drops CO). For ages 2-5, Thyme would be diluted 3x the label recommendation, which is 1:12 (1 drop EO:12 drops CO). For ages 5-10, Thyme would be diluted 2x the recommendation, which is 1:8 (1 drop EO:8 drops CO). Most recipes below are diluted for ages 5-10.

Dilution Chart for Children
6 months – 2 Years = Dilute 4x the label recommendation
2 Years – 5 Years = Dilute 3x the label recommendation
5 Years – 10 Years = Dilute 2x the label recommendation

Fever – RB

3 drops Peppermint
Mix Peppermint in 1 tablespoon CO and apply under armpits, down spine and on bottom of feet. Wait 10 minutes and reapply if needed. May also use Lemon diluted in the same places. For ages 5-10.

Respiratory/Cold/Flu/Allergy Trio – RB

4 drops Lemon
4 drops Lavender
4 drops Peppermint
Add all to RB and top with CO. Apply to wrists and behind ears as needed. For ages 5-10.

Growing Pains Massage Oil Version #1 – Dropper Bottle

7 drops Lavender
7 drops Lemongrass
Add all to 10 ml dropper bottle, top with CO. Massage into areas of concern as needed. For ages 5-10.

Growing Pains Massage Oil Version #2 – Dropper Bottle

6 drops Copaiba
4 drops Lemongrass
4 drops Peppermint
Add to 10 ml dropper bottle and top with CO. Massage into areas of concern as needed. For ages 5-10.

Ouch! Oil – Dropper Bottle

4 drops Melaleuca Alternifolia
4 drops Lavender
4 drops Frankincense
2 drops Lemongrass
Add all to 10 ml dropper bottle, top with CO. Apply to cuts or scrapes as needed. For ages 5-10.

Tummy Aches – RB

4 drops Peppermint
3 drops Spearmint
3 drops Ginger
2 drops Tangerine

2 drops Lavender

Add all to RB and top with CO. Apply in clockwise circles over area of discomfort. For ages 5-10.

Teething Baby – Dropper Bottle

2 drops Copaiba or Frankincense

Add Copaiba or Frankincense to a 5 ml dropper bottle and top with CO. Apply directly to affected area. For ages 6 months-2 years.

Teething Child – Dropper Bottle

5 drops Clove

Top with CO in a 5 ml dropper bottle and massage tooth and gum area as needed. For ages 5-10.

Rashes – Dropper Bottle

6 drops Roman Chamomile

4 drops Lavender

4 drops Sandalwood

Add all in a 10 ml dropper bottle, top with CO, and apply to rash as needed. For ages 5-10.

Lice Prevention Version #1 – Spray

10 drops Melaleuca Alternifolia

10 drops Lavender

1 t Epsom Salt

8 T Distilled Water

In a 4 oz glass spray bottle, combine Epsom salt and essential oils, swirling to mix. Top with distilled water. Spritz daily in hair, on sweaters, bookbags, etc. for protection against lice. Add 1-2 drops per oz of Melaleuca Alternifolia to both shampoo and conditioner as additional prevention.

Lice Prevention Version #2 – Spray

8 drops Eucalyptus Globulus

8 drops Rosemary

6 drops Melaleuca Alternifolia

10 drops Jojoba

1 t Epsom Salt

8 T Distilled Water

In a 4 oz glass spray bottle, combine Epsom salt and essential oils, swirling to mix. Top with jojoba and distilled water. Spritz daily in hair, on sweaters, bookbags, etc. for protection against lice. Add 1-2 drops per oz of Melaleuca Alternifolia to both shampoo and conditioner as additional prevention.

Immunity Booster – RB

6 drops Antibacterial Blend [Recipe on page 19]

6 drops Melaleuca Alternifolia

2 drops Oregano

Top with CO. Rub on bottom of feet, down spine, and at back of neck daily. For ages 5-10.

Sleepy Time – RB

6 drops Roman Chamomile
3 drops Lavender
3 drops Bergamot
2 drops Cedarwood
Top with CO. Apply 30 minutes before bedtime. Use as needed on bottom of the feet, wrists or back of neck. For ages 5-10.

Anti-Anxiety/Calming – RB

4 drops Palmarosa
3 drops Cedarwood
3 drops Orange
2 drops Lavender
2 drops Ylang Ylang
Top with CO. Use as needed on bottom of the feet, wrists or back of neck. For ages 5-10.

No More Missing Mommy – RB

4 drops Vetiver
4 drops Frankincense
3 drops Cedarwood
3 drops Lavender
Top with CO. Use as needed on bottom of the feet, wrists or back of neck. For ages 5-10.

Grump Away – RB

4 drops Lavender
4 drops Copaiba
4 drops Vetiver
2 drops Cedarwood
Top with CO. Use as needed on bottom of the feet, wrists or back of neck. For ages 5-10.

Calming Blend – RB

8 drops Orange
3 drops Bergamot
3 drops Roman Chamomile
Top with CO. For children dealing with separation issues, I like to attach a label that says, "Wear over your heart while we are apart, to remind you how much you are loved!" For ages 5-10.

Peaceful Child Blend – RB

4 drops Vetiver
4 drops Ylang Ylang
2 drops Frankincense
2 drops Clary Sage

2 drops Marjoram
Top with CO. Use as needed on bottom of the feet, wrists or back of neck. For ages 5-10.

Essential Oil Scented Sidewalk Chalk – Tub

5 drops Essential Oil(s) of choice
1 C of Plaster of Paris
¾ C Water
¼ C Tempera Liquid Paint
1 Large Plastic Cup
1 Plastic Spoon
Silicone Mold
In a large plastic cup, mix water, tempera paint, and essential oil well. When mixed, quickly add Plaster of Paris. Mix completely as quickly as possible and pour into molds. Let harden in molds for 24 hours, then remove from molds and let it air dry completely for another 24 hours.

Therapeutic Playdough for Kids – Jar

10 drops Essential Oil(s) of choice: Peppermint to stimulate, Lemon to cleanse and focus, Orange to soothe, Lavender to calm - your favorite essential oils for their various properties will work.
1 C Flour
½ C Kosher Salt
2 T Cream of Tartar
1 T Vegetable Oil
1 C Water
Food Coloring
Mix together the flour, kosher salt, cream of tartar, oil, and water in a medium saucepan. Cook over low/medium heat, stirring. Once it begins to thicken, add the food coloring. Continue stirring until the mixture is much thicker and begins to gather around the spoon. Place the dough onto waxed paper or a plate to cool slightly. To add the oils, roll the playdough into a ball and make a well in the center. Add 10 drops of essential oil (or your desired amount) and knead it into the playdough to spread it. Store in airtight container until ready to play. Yields about 20 oz of playdough.

Scented Finger Paint – Jar

Essential Oil(s) of choice
1½ C Cold Water
1¼ C Hot Water
1 C Flour
2 T Kosher Salt
Food Coloring or Natural Dye
Combine the flour, kosher salt and cold water in a saucepan and whisk until smooth. Heat over medium heat and slowly add 1¼ cups of hot water. Stir continuously until it comes to a boil and thickens. Divide into different containers and stir until smooth. Allow to cool. Add 1 drop essential oil (Lavender, Orange, Lemon, etc.) and 4-5 drops of food coloring or natural dye, stirring well. Put airtight lids on containers when not in use.

Rice Heat Packs

Use small square or rectangular pieces of fabric cut to the same size. Place two squares on top of each other, and sew three sides together. Fill the heating pack approximately ⅔ full of rice, add a few drops of essential oil of choice, then sew the open end closed. To use the heat pack, simply warm it in the microwave for a few minutes before using it to soothe sore muscles, ease stomach cramps, etc. When the essential oil wears off, simply place a few more drops on the outside of the heat pack.

Baby Wipes – Tub

5 drops Lavender or Frankincense
1 Roll of Natural Paper Towels
2½ C Distilled Warm Water
2 T Unscented Mild Castile Soap
2 T Sweet Almond Oil

Cut the roll of paper towels in half using a serrated knife. Lay half of the roll out flat, removing the cardboard center. Place the paper towels in an airtight container, or if one is not available, lay them flat in a sealable bag. In a bowl, whisk all liquid ingredients, and when well-blended, pour onto the paper towels and seal the container or bag. Let the wipes sit overnight until liquid is absorbed. Keep covered and sealed until needed. Should wipes dry out in between uses, simply add a bit more distilled water.

Men

Essential Oil Scent Chart

Woodsy – Cypress, Sandalwood, Spruce, Pine, Fir, Cedarwood
Spicy – Black Pepper, Clove, Cardamom, Bay Leaf, Nutmeg, Ginger
Floral – Neroli, Ylang Ylang
Earthy – Patchouli, Spikenard, Vetiver
Citrus – Lemon, Orange, Tangerine, Bergamot, Lime
Balsamic – Frankincense, Myrrh

Aftershave Oils – Single Application

1 drop Idaho Balsam Fir, Idaho Blue Spruce or Cedarwood
Add essential oil to a dab of CO and apply as needed.

Rum Spice Aftershave – Bottle

5 drops Cinnamon Bark
4 drops Nutmeg
4 drops Orange
3 drops Rosemary
1 C Witch Hazel
½ C Jamaican Rum
½ C Aloe Vera Gel

1 T Vegetable Glycerin

¾ t Vanilla Extract

Using a funnel, add all ingredients into a 16 oz glass flip-top bottle. Close the bottle and shake gently to combine ingredients.

Cologne – Spray

15 drops Idaho Blue Spruce

5 drops Cedarwood

½ t Epsom Salt

1 t Witch Hazel

3 T Distilled Water

Add Epsom salt and essential oils in a 2 oz glass spray bottle. Swirl to mix. Add the essential oils and 1 teaspoon of witch hazel. Fill with distilled water and shake well before use.

Rosemary Mint Shaving Cream – Jar

10 drops Rosemary

5 drops Peppermint

⅓ C Shea Butter

⅓ C Coconut Oil

⅓ C Jojoba

In a double boiler, heat shea butter and coconut oil, stirring until melted. Remove from heat, cool slightly, and add remaining oils. Place in refrigerator to chill until solid, whip until light and airy, and store in two 8 oz glass jars.

Simple Homemade Shaving Cream – Jar

4 drops Cedarwood

4 drops Lavender

2 drops Lime

¼ C Sweet Almond Oil

¼ C of your preferred brand of All-Natural Conditioner

Combine all ingredients in a bowl, and whip with an electric mixer until light and airy. Store in a 4 oz glass jar.

Beard Softening Oil – Dropper Bottle

10 drops Bergamot

5 drops Patchouli

3 drops Cedarwood

3 drops Cardamom

10 ml Argan Oil

Add essential oils to a 10 ml dropper bottle. Top with argan oil. Use one dropper full for a soft, manageable beard.

Beard Oil – Dropper Bottle

9-15 drops Essential Oil of choice

1 t Hemp Seed Oil

1 t Argan Oil

Add essential oils of choice to a 10 ml dropper bottle. Top with hemp and sweet almond oils. Shake well before use. Use one dropper full for a soft, manageable beard.

Beard Balm – Jar

10-20 drops Essential Oils of choice, suggestions include:

    Sweet and Woodsy Essential Oil Blend

    8 drops Idaho Blue Spruce

    4 drops Frankincense

    2 drops Rosemary

    2 drops Bergamot

2 T Beeswax Pellets

2 T Jojoba

1 T Shea Butter

1 T Argan Oil

5 drops Vitamin E Oil

Heat beeswax, jojoba and shea butter in a double boiler. When completely melted, remove from heat. Quickly add all oils, give it one last stir, and immediately pour into a 4 oz glass jar. Let the balm solidify for at least two hours, stir well, then cover with a tight-fitting lid. (Helpful hint: circular metal tins as containers make a nice presentation for gifting.)

Migraine Remedy for Men – Capsule

4 drops Idaho Blue Spruce

Empty '00' Vegetable Capsules

Add essential oils to a size '00' empty vegetable capsule, top with CO and take orally.

Prostatitis – Single Application

2 drops Peppermint, Tsuga or Thyme

20 drops CO

Topical Application: Mix and apply to area between scrotum and anus twice daily.

Retention Method: Insert rectally. Retain for as long as possible once per day.

Oral administration – Capsule:

3 drops Oregano

3 drops Vetiver

3 drops Peppermint

Add essential oils to a size '00' empty vegetable capsule, top with CO and take orally.

Cover Scent Blend – Spray

10 drops Cedarwood

10 drops Pine

8 drops Idaho Balsam Fir
6 drops Myrrh
5 drops Vetiver
½ t Epsom Salt
3 T Distilled Water
Mix oils with Epsom salt in a 2 oz glass spray bottle. Swirl to mix. Top with distilled water. Use to help cover your scent while hunting, or to cover your tracks if you weren't.

Food and Beverage

Essential Oil Wolfberry Gummies

6 drops Orange
¼ C Juice (i.e. Organic Apple or fresh squeezed Orange Juice)
¼ C nutrient infused Wolfberry Juice
1¼ packets of Gelatin (or vegan gelatin substitute)
1½ T local Honey
Candy Molds
Whisk apple or orange juice and gelatin in a saucepan on low until gelatin is dissolved. Remove from heat. Whisk in honey, wolfberry drink and essential oil. Pour into molds and let cool, placing in refrigerator to speed the process. Pop out of mold and enjoy!

Oil Infused Apples

1 drop Cinnamon Bark
1 drop Lemon
1 Apple
Add essential oils to a bowl of water containing thinly sliced apples. Soak for 10 minutes and enjoy.

Sun-Dried Tomato Spread

2 drops Black Pepper
1 drop Basil
2 packages Cream Cheese, softened
1 Jar (6-8 oz) Sun-Dried Tomatoes
1 T fresh Basil, minced
3-4 Green Onions
½ t Sea Salt
Let the cream cheese set on counter for 30 minutes to soften. Dice the tomatoes, green onions and mince the Basil. Put everything in a bowl and blend well. Cover tightly and place in refrigerator for an hour to marry the flavors. Test the seasonings, modify if needed and serve with celery, carrots, or whole grain club crackers.

Grape Salad

2-3 drops Lemon or Essential Oil of choice

8 oz Sour Cream
8 oz Cream Cheese
½ C Sugar
1 T Vanilla Extract
2 lbs. Green Seedless Grapes
2 lbs. Red Seedless Grapes
2 C Pecans
1 Pint Strawberries, sliced

Blend cream cheese and sugar together with an electric mixer; add sour cream and vanilla, stirring well. Save a few pieces of fruit and pecans to garnish the top, then fold in all other ingredients, making sure to coat evenly. Cover tightly with plastic wrap and place in the refrigerator for an hour to allow the flavors time to marry. Garnish before serving. This recipe will feed 7-10 people.

Mediterranean Style Marinated Steak

2 drops Lemon
1 drop Black Pepper
1 drop Oregano
2 lb. Flat Iron Steak
¾ C Olive Oil
½ C Soy Sauce
1 T Red Wine Vinegar
1 clove Garlic, minced

Combine all ingredients in a gallon size sealable bag, remove as much air as possible, seal tightly and refrigerate 2-8 hours. After marinating, place on counter and allow to rest at room temperature for 30 minutes. Grill or pan roast as desired.

Roasted Cauliflower and Garlic Pods

3 drops Lemon
1 head Cauliflower
6 Cloves Garlic, unpeeled
2 T Balsamic Vinegar
2 T Olive Oil
½ T Coarse Sea Salt

Cut Cauliflower into bite size florets. Combine all ingredients in a large sealable bag, mixing well. Pour onto a lightly greased foil-lined baking sheet, and cook at 425°F for approximately 20 minutes.

Roasted Lemon Green Beans

3 drops Lemon
1 lb. Fresh Green Beans, trimmed
2 T Olive Oil
½ T Coarse Sea Salt
Optional: ½ t Garlic Powder
Fresh Ground Pepper

Preheat oven to 400°F. Spread green beans on a lightly greased foil-lined baking sheet, drizzle with olive oil and sprinkle with salt and pepper. Roast approximately 15 minutes until tender-crisp. Place green beans in a serving bowl, add Lemon, and toss. Serve warm, adding additional salt and pepper if needed.

Orange Creamsicle Cheesecake Dip

4-6 drops Orange
16 oz Cream Cheese, softened
6 T Granulated Sugar
⅔ C Vanilla Greek Yogurt
2 t Vanilla Extract
¼ t Sea Salt
In a medium mixing bowl, beat cream cheese and sugar for 2 minutes, until fluffy. Add the yogurt and whip for 2 more minutes. Add vanilla, Orange and sea salt; beat for a final 2 minutes until smooth and creamy. Serve with assorted fruits, cookies or pretzels. Yields approximately 3 cups.

Citrus Fruit Dip

2 drops Lemon
2 drops Essential Oil of choice
8 oz Cream Cheese, softened
1 Jar (8 oz) Marshmallow Cream
1 t Vanilla Extract
Place cream cheese and marshmallow cream in a mixing bowl and blend well. Add vanilla extract, 2 drops of Lemon and 2 drops of essential oil of choice. Lemon and Lime are delicious together, you can add Orange or Tangerine, the options are many! Serve with a fresh cut fruit tray or platter of cookies. Makes approximately 16 oz.

Lemon Bars

Crust:
2 C Flour
½ C Sugar
1 C Butter
¼ t Sea Salt

Filling:
3 drops Lemon
4 Eggs
6 T Flour
1½ C Sugar
1 t Baking Powder
Pinch of Salt
½ C Water
½ C Lemon Juice

1 T Powdered Sugar

Optional: Lemon Zest

Preheat oven to 350°F. To make crust mix flour, sugar, and salt in a medium size bowl; cut in the butter until the dough reaches a fine crumb consistency. Press dough into the bottom of a lightly greased 9"x13" pan. Bake for 20 minutes until golden brown. Beat eggs in a large mixing bowl, and in a separate dish stir together flour, sugar, baking powder and salt. Add eggs to mixture, stirring until smooth. Gradually stir in lemon juice, water and essential oil. Pour mixture over baked crust and return to the oven, baking for 30 minutes or until set. Cool completely and sift powdered sugar on top. Garnish with zest if desired. (Helpful hint: can substitute orange juice and orange essential oil to make Orange Bars.)

Lemon Drop Cream Cheese Cookies

15 drops Lemon

2 oz Cream Cheese

6 T unsalted Butter, softened

1 Egg

½ t Vanilla Extract

1¾ C Flour

¾ C White Sugar

¼ C Powdered Sugar

¼ t Sea Salt

¼ t Baking Powder

¼ t Baking Soda

1 T Powdered Sugar to dust tops of cookies

Heat the oven to 350°F. Cream butter, cream cheese and sugars together until smooth. Add the essential oil, vanilla extract and eggs, continuing to mix. In a separate bowl, mix together dry ingredients. Combine the dry and wet ingredients and mix well. Scoop cookies onto a baking sheet and bake for 9-10 minutes. Remove from oven and dust with powdered sugar. (Helpful hint: don't worry, the dough will taste stronger than the finished product!)

Dark Chocolate Peppermint Truffles

5 drops Peppermint

1½ T Shortening

¼ C Coconut Milk Creamer (or regular Coconut Milk)

1 C Dark Chocolate Chips

1 t Vanilla Extract

¼ C Unsweetened Cocoa Powder

Melt the shortening over low heat in a small saucepan. Add the coconut milk or creamer increasing the heat to medium, and barely bring to a boil, stirring occasionally. Remove saucepan from heat and stir in chocolate chips and vanilla extract. Stir vigorously until the mixture is smooth and glossy. Add Peppermint, and transfer to a large mixing bowl and refrigerate for approximately 1 hour, until hardened but pliable. Soften using the paddle attachment of a mixer for about 20 seconds on low speed. Using a teaspoon or melon baller, scoop chocolate and form balls 1" in diameter using cool, dry hands and very light pressure. Place on waxed paper. (Helpful hint: If your hands start to get too warm or the chocolate starts to soften, refrigerate the chocolates for a few minutes and start again.) When you are finished forming the balls, place them in the refrigerator for approximately 15 minutes. Remove truffles from the refrigerator and toss them in cocoa powder to finish. May be stored in a sealed container in the refrigerator for up to two weeks. Best when served at room temperature.

Peppermint Patties

10 drops Peppermint
1 lb Powdered Sugar
4 oz Cream Cheese, softened
6 oz semi-sweet Chocolate Chips

Using an electric mixer, slowly add the powdered sugar to the cream cheese. When blended, add Peppermint, stirring well. Roll dough into teaspoon size balls and place on a baking sheet lined with wax paper. Create a small "bowl" or indention in the top of each ball using a ¼ teaspoon measuring spoon or your little finger. Cover tray with plastic wrap and let firm in the refrigerator for a few hours. When peppermints are firm, melt chocolate according to package directions. Fill a piping bag, or a plastic bag with the corner snipped off, with melted chocolate. Fill each peppermint bowl/indention with chocolate, and let cool. Refrigerate in an airtight container until ready to serve.

Ginger Bread People

2 drops Ginger
1 drop Cinnamon Bark
3 C Flour
1 t Baking Soda
¼ t Sea Salt
¾ C Butter or Coconut Oil
¾ C firmly packed Brown or Coconut Sugar
½ C Molasses
1 Egg or Vegan Egg Substitute
1 t Vanilla Extract

In a medium bowl, whisk together dry ingredients and set aside. In a larger bowl, mix together butter or coconut oil and sugar until light and airy. Beat in remaining wet ingredients. Gradually add flour mixture until dough forms, being careful not to overmix. Press dough into a flat disk, cover with plastic wrap, and refrigerate overnight or at minimum 4 hours. Preheat oven to 350°F. Roll dough out ¼" thick on a clean and lightly floured countertop. Use cookie cutters to cut desired shapes. Place 1" apart on ungreased cookie sheet and bake 8–10 minutes or until edges are just beginning to brown. Cool completely and decorate as desired.

Lavender and Honey Lemonade

3 drops Lavender
2 drops Lemon
6 Lemons
2 Limes
¾ C local Honey
2 C Water

In a medium saucepan bring water to a boil, and add honey. Stir well to dissolve, and place saucepan in the refrigerator to cool. Juice 4 lemons and 1 lime, adding juice and pulp to a 1 gallon pitcher. Slice the remaining 2 lemons and lime, adding them to the pitcher for decoration. Add essential oils and honey mixture, stirring well. Top with water and chill until ready to serve.

Citrus Fruity Drink Mix

5 drops Lemon
5 drops Orange (or other Citrus Oil of choice)
1 bag of Frozen Fruit Mix
1 gallon of Water
½ of a fresh Lemon for garnish
Combine ingredients in a gallon size pitcher, mix well, and serve over ice.

Citrus Sangria

5 drops Orange
5 drops Grapefruit
3 drops Lemon
3 bottles Red Wine
1 C fresh-squeezed Orange Juice
1 C fresh-squeezed Grapefruit Juice
½ C Brandy or Rum
2 T local Honey
2 Apples, cut into 2" chunks
2 Oranges, cut into 1" round slices
1 Lemon, cut into 1" round slices
1 C Seltzer Water
1 pint Strawberries for garnish
Mix wine, honey, juices and Brandy or Rum in a large pitcher, stirring until honey is dissolved. Add fruit and refrigerate overnight. Just before serving, add essential oils and seltzer water. Garnish with fresh strawberries.

Household Cleaning

All Purpose Cleaning – Spray

10 drops Lemon
3 drops Melaleuca Alternifolia
5 drops Rosemary
5 drops Orange
2 C Distilled Water
2 T White Vinegar
Combine all ingredients in a 16 oz glass spray bottle. Shake well before use.

Lemon Fresh – Spray

10 drops Lemon
8 T Witch Hazel
8 T Distilled Water
Combine all in an 8 oz glass spray bottle. Shake well, and use as needed to help disinfect surfaces or provide an aromatic boost.

Surface Sanitizer – Spray

30 drops Antibacterial Blend [Recipe on page 19]
2 t Witch Hazel
8 T Distilled Water
Combine witch hazel and essential oils in a 4 oz glass spray bottle. Shake well before use.

Dusting Spray and Polish – Spray

8 drops Orange
4 drops Cedarwood
4 drops Lemon
¼ C Distilled Water
½ T Castile Soap
½ t Olive Oil
Add oils to a 10 oz glass spray bottle, swirling to combine. Add the castile soap, mixing well, followed by the water. Shake well before use.

Homemade Citrus Dish Soap – Pump Jar

5 drops Lemon
5 drops Lemongrass
3 drops Orange
1 C Liquid Castile Soap
⅓ C Distilled Water
1 t Vegetable Glycerin
½ t Sea Salt
Add sea salt to a 12 oz glass jar. Add essential oils and swirl the jar to mix. Add water, close the jar, and shake until the salt is dissolved. Add vegetable glycerin and castile soap. Shake well before use.

Sunshine Sink Scrub – Single Application

5 drops Lemon
1 drop Orange
¼ C Baking Soda
Pour baking soda into a pile directly in the sink. Add essential oils on top. Dampen 2 fingers and stir into a paste. With a damp sponge, thoroughly clean the sink. This removes grease, grime and black marks, and smells wonderful while you clean.

Tub Scrub – Jar

5 drops Clove
5 drops Orange
½ C Liquid Castile Soap
½ C Baking Soda

In an 8 oz glass jar, mix castile soap and baking soda to form a paste. Add essential oils and stir well. To use, apply a small amount to a sponge or cloth, and be sure to keep the jar sealed when not in use. (Helpful hint: Melaleuca Alternifolia, Rosemary, Lavender, Lemon and Peppermint all make wonderful substitutions in this recipe.)

Laminate Floor Cleaning – Spray

3 drops Lemon
3 drops Clove or Peppermint
⅔ C Alcohol
⅔ C Vinegar
⅔ C Water
3 drops of your preferred brand dish soap

Combine all ingredients in a 16 oz glass spray bottle. Shake well before use.

Carpet Freshener Tip

Add 3 drops of your favorite essential oil directly to your vacuum filter before using.

Carpet and Mattress Freshener – Sprinkle Jar

10 drops Lemon, Lemongrass or Melaleuca Alternifolia
3 drops Peppermint
2 C Cornstarch or Baking Soda

Thoroughly combine ingredients in a 16 oz glass jar. Cap tightly and let sit for 24 hours. To use, lightly sprinkle carpet or mattress and vacuum after 30 minutes. (Helpful hint: I make this in a glass jar with holes drilled in the metal lid as a makeshift shaker. When I am not using it, I cover the top with plastic wrap and a rubber band to preserve the freshness.)

Room Sprays and Pillow Spritzers – Spray

10-20 drops Essential Oil(s) of choice
½ t Sea Salt
¾ C Water
¼ C Witch Hazel

In an 8 oz glass spray bottle, add sea salt and essential oils, swirling to mix. Top with water and witch hazel. Shake well before use. The following are popular spritzer combinations, let your nose be your guide!

> Minty Citrus Twist 4 drops Peppermint, 4 drops Orange, 1 T Vanilla Extract
> Sweet Lavender 8 drops Lavender, 1 T Vanilla Extract
> Summer Citrus 3 drops Orange, 3 drops Lemon, 3 drops Lime, 3 drops Grapefruit
> Cozy Holiday 3 drops Orange, 3 drops Cassia, 3 drops Clove, 1 T Vanilla Extract

Sweet Orange 6 drops Orange, 4 drops Lemon, 1 T Vanilla Extract
Evergreen 3 drops Blue Spruce, 4 drops Pine, 4 drops Cedarwood
Welcome Fall 4 drops Cardamom, 4 drops Clove, 2 drops Orange, 1 drop Nutmeg

Household Laundry

Liquid Laundry Detergent – Jug

20 drops Essential Oil(s) of choice
¼ of 5 oz bar of Fels-Naptha soap, grated
2 C Water
¼ C Borax
¼ C Super Washing Soda
½ C of your preferred brand of All-Natural Household Cleaner
In a saucepan on low heat, combine soap, water, borax, and super washing soda until powders are dissolved. Remove from heat and add ½ cup of your preferred brand of all-natural household cleaner and 20 drops of essential oil of choice. Pour mixture into a 1 gallon jug and top with 64 oz of water. Let it sit overnight before first use.

Powdered Laundry Detergent – Jar

25 drops Essential Oil of choice
1 C Borax
1 C Super Washing Soda
5 oz bar of Fels-Naptha Soap, grated
In a large bowl, combine and mix dry ingredients. Add essential oil of choice, and finish mixing well. Pour into a 20 oz glass jar or container. Use 2 tablespoons per load of laundry.

Whitener and Brightener – Single Application

2 drops Lemon
¼ C Hydrogen Peroxide
Mix and add to the bleach compartment of your washing machine, or directly to the water. Launder as usual. Treat Hydrogen Peroxide like bleach, and do not use it on your colored laundry.

Oxygen Bleach Paste – Single Application

2 drops Lemon
1 T Hydrogen Peroxide
1 T Washing Soda
Combine in a small bowl. The consistency should be a dry paste, not powdery. Add a little water to the bowl before putting the bleach in the detergent dispenser or directly into the washing machine water. After the ingredients are mixed, they lose their effectiveness in a few hours, so use right away.

General Stain – Spray

6 drops Lemon
½ C Distilled Water
2 T Borax

In an 8 oz glass spray bottle, combine all ingredients. Shake thoroughly. Spray directly on stain and launder as usual. Store up to 1 month.

Melaleuca Alternifolia Stain – Stick

4 drops Melaleuca Alternifolia
2.5 oz bar of Castile Soap
1 T Distilled Water

Grate soap. Place in microwave safe bowl and add the water. Melt on low heat in 30 second intervals for about a minute and a half, stirring at 30 second intervals. When melted, let it cool approximately 5 minutes and stir in Melaleuca Alternifolia. Pour in a clean 2.5 oz container with a push up bottom. Store in a cool place for up to 6 months.

Basic Fabric Softener – Jar

10 drops Essential Oil of choice
3 C Vinegar
¼ C Isopropyl Alcohol

Mix all ingredients together and store in a 26 oz glass jar. To use, add ¼ cup directly to washing machine or into the fabric softener dispensing cup.

Advanced Lemon Clove Fabric Softener – Jug

20 drops Lemon
10 drops Clove
64 oz White Vinegar
1 C Baking Soda

Optional: 1 C of All-Natural Hair Conditioner for a thicker consistency and "store bought" look.
Pour vinegar in a large bowl. SLOWLY whisk in baking soda. If using, add conditioner and blend well, followed by the essential oils. Store in a 64 oz container. Shake well before use. Add a ¼ cup directly to washing machine water or into the fabric softener dispensing cup.

Dryer Sheets – Jar

10 drops Essential Oil(s) of choice
1 C Vinegar
Thin Cotton Cloths cut to approximately 6"x6"

Put cloths in a 32 oz glass jar and top with vinegar and essential oils of choice. Shake well. Pull a cloth out as needed and add into dryer with your wet clothing. This helps to soften laundry, yet leaves no smell of vinegar behind. When removing the cloth from the dryer, simply add it back into your jar.

Outdoors

Garden Insect Deterrent – Spray

20-24 drops Essential Oil(s) of choice
1 t of your preferred brand all-natural Liquid Soap
2 C Water
Add soap, essential oils of choice and water to a 16 oz glass spray bottle. Shake well before use. Spray around the garden to deter insects. Not all insects are repelled by the same essential oil, but a few popular garden pests along with some of their repellants are listed below:

- Ants – Peppermint
- Aphids – Peppermint, Spearmint
- Caterpillars – Peppermint
- Chiggers – Lavender, Lemongrass, Thyme
- Fleas – Lavender, Lemongrass, Peppermint
- Flies – Peppermint, Rosemary, Lavender, Sage, Patchouli
- Gnats – Patchouli
- Mosquitos – Eucalyptus Radiata, Peppermint, Lemongrass, Lemon, Clove
- Roaches – Cypress, Peppermint
- Slugs – Cedarwood
- Spiders – Peppermint, Spearmint
- Ticks – Peppermint, Geranium, Thyme, Lavender, Lemongrass, Melaleuca Alternifolia

Mosquito and Bug Repellant – Spray

15-20 drops Essential Oil(s) of choice
3 T Distilled Water
1 t Vegetable Glycerin
2 t Witch Hazel or Vodka
½ t Epsom Salt
In a 4 oz glass spray bottle add Epsom salt and essential oils of choice. Swirl so that oils are absorbed by the salt. Add all other ingredients and shake well before use. Ideas for blends are as follows, and it is a good idea to modify chosen oils based on the relevant insects at hand (See Chart under Garden Insect Deterrent – Spray).

Floral 8 drops Geranium, 5 drops Lavender, 5 drops Rosemary, 2 drops Patchouli
Dusky 10 drops Lavender, 6 drops Cedarwood, 4 drops Patchouli
Fresh 12 drops Grapefruit, 5 drops Peppermint, 3 drops Eucalyptus
Outdoors 10 drops Rosemary, 6 drops Cedarwood, 4 drops Cinnamon Bark
Clean 10 drops Melaleuca Alternifolia, 6 drops Thyme, 4 drops Grapefruit

Bug Off – Jar

10 drops Peppermint
10 drops Lavender
8 T Coconut Oil

In a 4 oz glass jar, combine ingredients and blend well. Before going outdoors where pests are an issue, apply cream over exposed areas. You can also melt and whip this recipe based on personal preference using the double boiler method. (Helpful hint: there are more lightweight carrier oils that might be a better summertime fit based on geography, including aloe vera gel and sweet almond or avocado oil.)

Insect Repellant Version #1 – Diffuser

2 drops Lemongrass
2 drops Melaleuca Alternifolia
2 drops Eucalyptus Radiata
1 drop Rosemary

Insect Repellant Version #2 – Diffuser

3 drops Citronella
2 drops Spearmint
1 drop Lemongrass
1 drop Peppermint

Insect Repellant Version #3 – Diffuser

3 drops Melaleuca Alternifolia
2 drops Rosemary
1 drop Thyme
1 drop Lavender

Chicken Coop Deodorizing – Spray

25 drops Lemon
1 C White Vinegar
1 C Water

Add ingredients to a 16 oz glass spray bottle. Top with 1 cup white vinegar and 1 cup water. Shake well before use. Use for cleaning nests, roosting bars, and general area where your chickens live and play - if you're like me, that's your garage ☺

Comedogenic Ratings

0 – Will not clog pores
1 – Low
2 – Moderately Low
3 – Moderate
4 – Relatively High
5 – High

There are many Carrier Oil options, all of which have a different impact on your skin. Below are listed various CO options, along with their comedogenic ratings. Comedogenic refers to the tendency to cause or aggravate acne.

Oils

Almond Oil – 2
Apricot Kernel Oil – 2
Avocado Oil – 2
Camphor – 2
Castor Oil – 1
Cocoa Butter – 4
Coconut Butter – 4
Coconut Oil – 4
Corn Oil – 3
Cotton Seed Oil – 3
Evening Primrose Oil – 2
Grapeseed Oil – 2
Hazelnut Oil – 2
Hemp Seed Oil – 0
Mineral Oil – 0
Mink Oil – 3
Olive Oil – 2
Onomethyl Ether – 0
Peanut Oil – 2
Petrolatum – 0
Safflower Oil – 0

Sandalwood Seed Oil - 2
Sesame Oil – 2
Shark Liver Oil – 3
Shea Butter – 0
Soybean Oil – 3
Sunflower Oil – 0
Wheat Germ Oil - 5

Waxes

Beeswax – 2
Candelilla Wax – 1
Carnuba Wax – 1
Ceresin Wax – 0
Emulsifying Wax – 2
Jojoba – 2
Lanolin Wax – 1
Sulfated Jojoba – 3

Botanicals

Algae Extract – 5
Aloe Vera Gel – 0
Calendula – 1

Carrageenans – 5
Chamomile – 2
Chamomile Extract – 0
Cold Pressed Aloe – 0
Red Algae – 5

Vitamins & Herbs

Ascorbic Acid – 0
Black Walnut Extract – 0
Vitamin E Oil – 2
Vitamin A Palmitate – 2
Panthenol – 0

Minerals

Algin – 4
Colloidal Sulphur – 3
Flowers of Sulphur – 0
Potassium Chloride – 5
Precipitated Sulphur – 0
Sodium Chloride (Salt) – 5
Talc – 1
Zinc Stearate – 0

Bibliography and Works Consulted

Breedlove, Greta. *The Herbal Home Spa. Naturally Refreshing Wraps. Rubs, Lotions, Masks, Oils and Scrubs.* North Adams, MA: Storey Publishing, 1998.

Dugliss-Wesselman, Stacey. *The Home Apothecary. Cold Spring Apothecary's Cookbook of Hand-Crafted Remedies and Recipes for the Hair, Skin, Body & Home.* Beverly, MA: Quarry Books, 2013.

Essential Oils Desk Reference, Third Edition. Lehi, UT: Essential Science Publishing, 2006.

Essential Oils Desk Reference, Sixth Edition. Lehi, UT: Life Science Publishing, 2015.

Higley, Connie & Alan. *Quick Reference Guide for Using Essential Oils.* Spanish Fork, UT: Abundant Health, 2014.

Keller, Erich. *Aromatherapy Handbook for Beauty, Hair and Skin Care.* Rochester, VT: Healings Arts Press, 1992.

Maria, Donna. *Making Aromatherapy Creams & Lotions: 101 Natural Formulas to Revitalize & Nourish Your Skin.* North Adams, MA: Storey Publishing, 2000.

National Association for Holistic Aromatherapy. www.naha.org. Raleigh, NC: 2017.

Reybern, Debra. *Gentle Babies, Essential Oils and Natural Remedies for Pregnancy, Childbirth, Infants and Young Children.* Revised Fifth Edition. Bartlesville, OK: Growing Healthy Homes, LLC, 2014.

Schnaubelt, Kurt, Ph.D. *The Healing Intelligence of Essential Oils. The Science of Advanced Aromatherapy.* Rochester, VT: Healing Arts Press, 2011.

Shutes, Jade. "Foundations of Aromatherapy Course" offered by The School for Aromatic Studies, 2016.

Shutes, Jade. "French Aromatherapy Course" offered by The School for Aromatic Studies, 2016.

Stewart, D. *Chemistry of Essential Oils Made Simple.* Marble Hill, MO: Care Publications, 2005.

Wormwood, Valerie Ann. *Aromatherapy for the Healthy Child: More than 300 Natural, Non-Toxic, and Fragrant Essential Oil Blends.* Novato, CA: New World Library, 2000.

Wormwood, Valerie Ann. *The Complete Book of Essential Oils and Aromatherapy.* Novato, CA: New World Library, 2016.

Young, D. Gary. *Essential Oils Integrative Medical Guide. Building Immunity, Increasing Longevity, and Enhancing Mental Performance with Therapeutic-Grade Essential Oils.* Lehi, UT: Life Science Publishing, 2013.

MY NOTES & RECIPES

As always, just holler if you need me ♡ Brandy

Made in the USA
Middletown, DE
10 November 2017